THE RESISTANCE BAND WORKOUT

John Edward Kennett

p

This is a Parragon Book
First published in 2006

Parragon
Queen Street House
4 Queen Street
Bath BA1 1HE, UK

ISBN: 1-40548-632-5
Printed in China

Created and produced by the Bridgewater Book Company Ltd
Photography: Ian Parsons
Hair and make-up stylist: Johan van der Merwe
Models: Katie Lawrie and Kevin Dixon
Illustrations: John Woodcock

The publisher would like to thank the following for permission to
reproduce copyright material: Brooke Fasani/Corbis (page 6) and
Ben Welsh/zefa/Corbis (page 7).

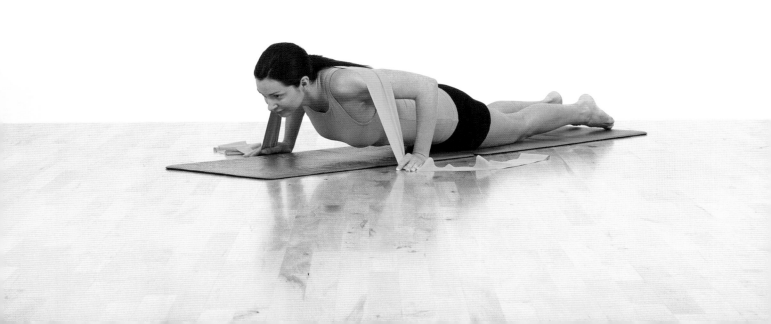

contents

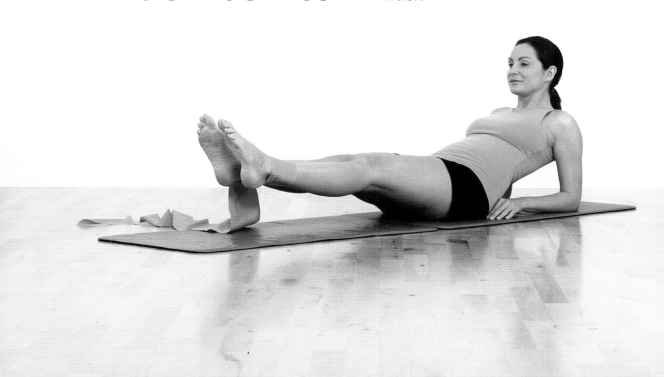

Resistance bands are amazing fitness tools. Their ability to improve your fitness and your strength, develop your muscle speed and stamina, and increase your body's mobility seems almost too good to be true for such simple objects and were seldom used by anyone other than top sports people. However, now resistance bands are starting to get the attention that they deserve, and with this book you will discover everything you need to know about using them.

With the assistance of this book you can build strength, speed and muscle stamina, decrease body fat, improve your flexibility and balance, and exercise and strengthen specific muscles that machines would miss. You can achieve your goal with a combination of resistance band exercises and a positive attitude that motivates you to keep up a consistent programme. You can exercise just about anywhere, it does not depend on the weather, and it is inexpensive. With this insightful book, the resistance band is no longer a secret.

Many people want to get fit and take up a sport – tennis, golf, football, cycling, swimming, skiing – in order to become fit. In doing so, though, they may soon suffer injuries that prevent them from pursuing the enjoyment of sport and the fundamental physiological and psychological health benefits that fitness gives them. Thus, it is not about playing a sport to become fit – it is about becoming fit in order to play and enjoy sport.

Research proves that resistance band training provides as much benefit in fitness and strength gains as those achieved on cumbersome and expensive weight-training equipment. The reason is simple – as the elastic band is stretched, so resistance increases, providing progressive stimulus to your muscles.

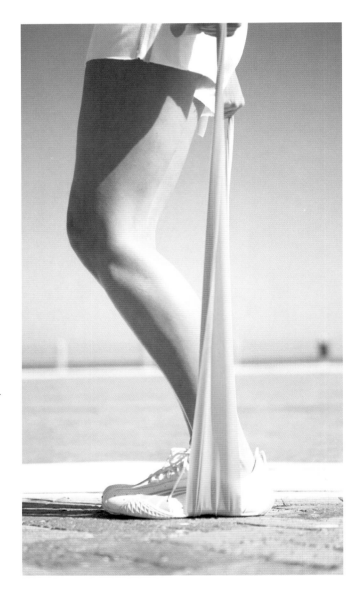

introduction

This book will guide you through some of the fundamental principles of exercise, teaching you how to prepare your body and motivate your mind to ensure you attain and maintain your desired results using resistance bands. You will gain an insight into how specific body types react to different resistance band exercises. You will learn that stretching is not warming up and warming up is not stretching, as well as the importance of a warm-down after you have exercised. You will be able to determine the correct percentage of your maximum heart rate within which to exercise, enabling you to lose body fat, increase your fitness or build muscle strength, or a combination of all three. This will enable you to choose and combine the resistance band exercises into a routine best suited to your body type and your desired outcome.

Until recently, resistance bands were mostly used in remedial physiotherapy, enabling patients to recover range of motion, strength and stability after injury. Knowledge of sports science has grown over recent years, and top sports people now utilize resistance band training to improve their performance. If you work with the resistance band, you can gain advantages in your fitness exercise regime and chosen sport.

CAUTION

Consult your health advisor before embarking on any new fitness programme, especially if you suffer from or have a history of high blood pressure or heart conditions.

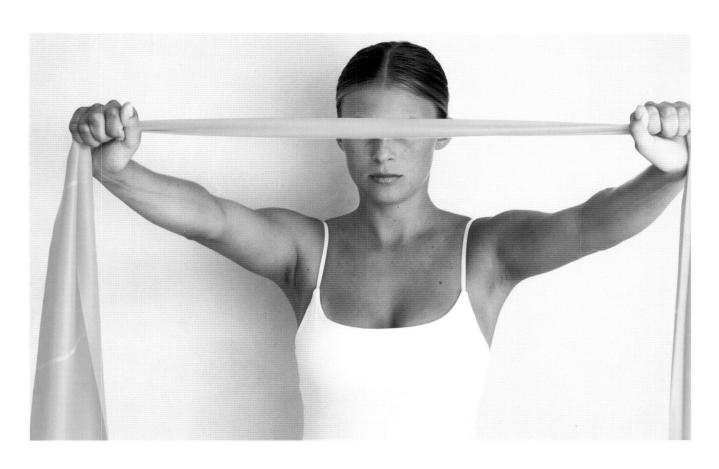

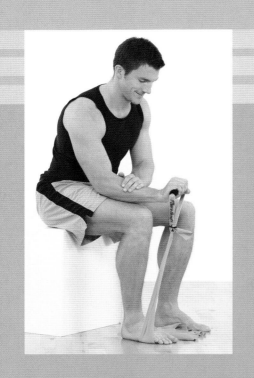
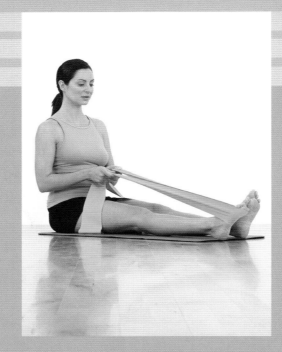
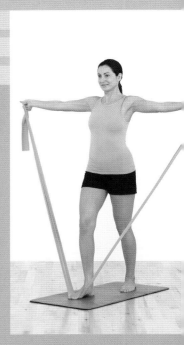

1
resistance band

Resistance band training offers you a number of benefits, and in this chapter you will learn how and why resistance bands work simply and effectively. You will discover the fundamental principles of exercise as practised by top sports people and dancers. Exercising within a specific heart-rate range, with an understanding of how body type enters into the equation, will empower you to decide which type of resistance band exercise suits your needs. You will also learn how you can maintain your consistency with exercise and enjoy the thrill of knowing that resistance band exercises can change your body, motivating you to reach your desired goal.

From beginners to seasoned athletes, we can all benefit by adding resistance bands and resistance tubes to our training programmes. There are many elastic band resistance products on the market, most developed from the two basic options of the resistance band and the resistance tube. Neither differs from the other in principle, concept or mechanics. In general, all the exercises can be done with either bands or tubing, depending upon your preference, and, unless specified, the use of the resistance band is identical to the resistance tube.

Resistance band training is simple: the more the elastic band is stretched, the more the resistance increases, and likewise, the band will contract as the force decreases. Neither type of elastic resistance relies on gravity, unlike most exercise machines and the classic free weights such as the dumb-bell; instead, resistance is dependent upon how far the resistance band is stretched, and continuously and increasingly places demands on your muscle as it contracts throughout the whole range of motion.

Both bands and tubing come in different lengths and many resistance levels. The bands or tubes are colour-coded according to their resistance levels. Different manufacturers use different colour schemes for their bands and tubes, but generally both the colour and resistance of the band or tube start light and progress through to darker colours, which represent increased resistance.

The possibilities of resistance bands are limited only by your imagination. They allow you to move more freely and achieve a greater range of motion than machines, which control where you start and stop. This allows you to create resistance from any direction – high overhead, below from floor level, or to the side, for example. By adjusting your angle of movement, moving the fixed point higher or lower, several exercises can be combined. Resistance bands allow you to imitate movements that you do in real life and exercise muscles that machines miss. Many different exercises can be performed with a single resistance band.

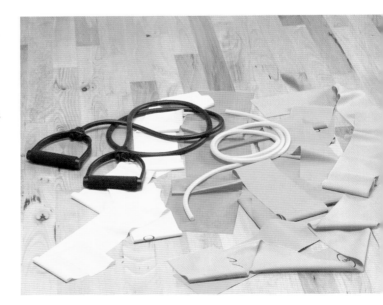

how resistance bands work

Resistance band exercising will assist in strengthening the muscles involved in respiration, facilitating the flow of air in and out of your lungs; aid in strengthening the heart, to improve its pumping efficiency and reduce your resting heart rate; tone the muscles throughout your body, which can improve your overall circulation and reduce blood pressure; and increase the number of red blood cells in your body, improving oxygen transportation.

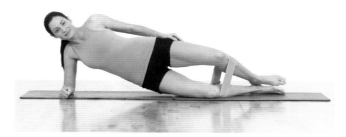

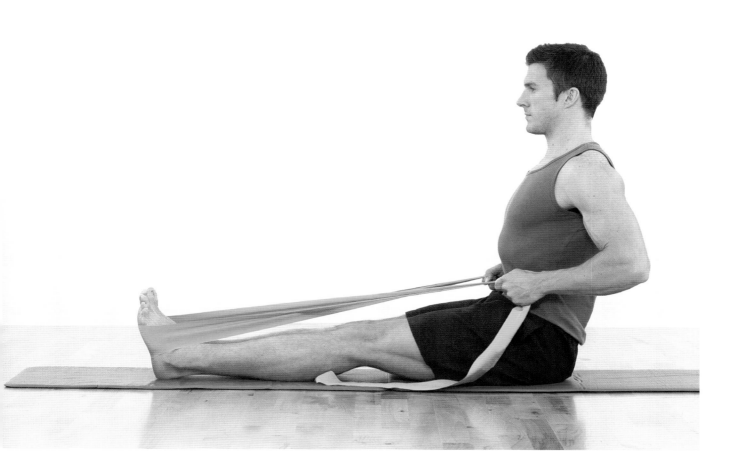

When working with resistance bands, it is extremely useful to have an understanding of basic anatomy. This makes it much easier to appreciate the many positive effects that training with resistance bands can have on different parts of the body.

Muscles and bones are collectively called the musculoskeletal system. Bones give structural and postural support to the body in conjunction with the muscles' ability to contract, enabling movement. The mechanical stresses imposed by resistance band exercises can improve bone condition. It has been shown in studies that where these stresses are applied on the skeleton the most, more mineral salts are deposited and more collagen fibres are produced, causing both the density and also the size of the bone to increase.

Bones are linked together via joints, which can be fixed, slightly movable or free:

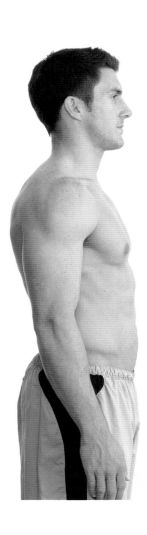

• Fixed, or fibrous, joints, such as the suture type found in the skull, bind the bones tightly together with fibrous connective tissue, permitting no movement between them.

• Slightly movable, or cartilaginous, joints, such as the pads of cartilage found in between the vertebrae of the spine, move by compression of the cartilage.

• Freely movable, or synovial, joints are of five different types:

1 Ball and socket joints, such as the hip and shoulder joints, are the most movable of all joints, allowing movement of limbs in many different directions.

2 Hinge joints, such as the knee and elbow, move in one directional plane only.

3 Gliding joints, such as the carpal bones in the hand and the tarsal bones in the foot, allow the bones to glide against each other and are the least movable of this type.

basic anatomy

4   Pivot joints allow a rotary movement about one axis, such as the first two cervical vertebrae, the atlas and axis, which allow the head to rotate.

5   Saddle joints are found only in the thumbs and provide movement about two axes, similar to a ball and socket joint, enabling the thumb to oppose the index finger.

Bones, tendons and ligaments are not able to make your body move – only muscles can do this. Varying in size and in shape, there are three types of muscle tissue which have different purposes:

•   Involuntary muscles, known as smooth muscles, differ from other muscle types in structure and function. Smooth muscles are found within the 'walls' of hollow organs such as blood vessels and the bladder and work automatically. Regular exercise with a resistance band can develop this muscle type, improving the muscles' efficiency.

•   Cardiac muscle exists only in the heart. It is myogenic, meaning that it stimulates its own contraction without a requisite electrical impulse. The resistance band exercises and workout routines will effectively exercise your heart, enabling it to work more efficiently.

•   Skeletal muscles, or voluntary muscles, are generally consciously controlled. Composed of a group of specialized strands of elastic tissues, bound together in bundles and contained in a sheath called fasculi, they combine to form the muscle belly. The ends of these bundles extend to form a tendon that attaches to other parts of the body; usually one end, the head or origin, is attached to a relatively stationary bone and the other end, the insertion, is attached across a joint to another bone. Muscles with two heads are known as the biceps, three heads

the triceps and four as the quadriceps. Working out with a resistance band can strengthen, lengthen and improve both your muscles' endurance and flexibility.

Skeletal muscles contain two types of muscle fibres. Type I 'slow twitch' fibres are good for endurance and are slow to tire. High repetition, low intensity resistance band exercise will stimulate and increase the proliferation of these fibres. Type II 'fast twitch' fibres are divided into type IIa for great strength, lasting over modest periods, and type IIb, also used for short bursts of speed and power but tiring even faster. Low repetition, high intensity resistance band exercise will build fast twitch muscle fibres.

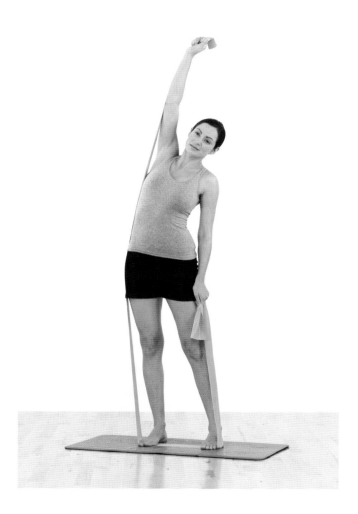

The muscles

For a muscle to contract it needs large amounts of energy and a message to be sent from the brain to initiate its movement. The body's energy is provided by a compound called adenosine triphosphate (ATP), which is made in muscle cells. Muscles have a store of energy generating ATP for about 10 seconds of exercise before depleting. The muscle will then convert ATP from carbohydrate that is stored in the form of glycogen. Waste products are created, such as lactic acid, which the body removes from the muscles to prevent build-up.

Each muscle fibre is innervated by a nerve called a motor neuron. A single motor neuron supplies many muscle fibres and is known as a motor unit. The nervous and muscular systems communicate via the neuromuscular junction. Here the muscle fibre is triggered by a nerve impulse having to bridge the gap between the muscle fibre and nerve ending. This happens indirectly by the secretion of a neurotransmitter called acetylcholine. Depending upon the muscle, a single motor neuron can innervate from one to many hundreds of muscle fibres.

All the body's movements involve the action of more than one muscle. The muscle primarily responsible for movement becomes known as the agonist. As it contracts, the opposing muscle, called the antagonist, relaxes to allow movement. For example, when flexing the elbow, the biceps brachii muscle acts as the agonist by contracting. The triceps brachii is the antagonist. The antagonist can also contract at the same time as the agonist, to control or slow down a movement.

By becoming familiar with the muscles that make up your body, you will become more familiar with the muscles that you are working, making it easier to feel and visualize which exercises are helping you to make the improvements you desire.

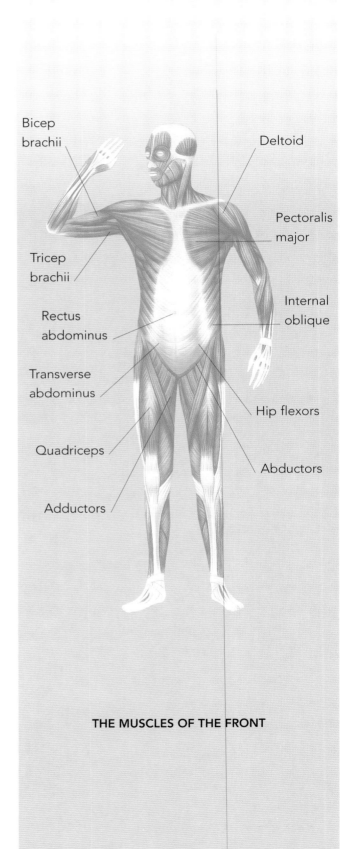

Bicep brachii

Deltoid

Pectoralis major

Tricep brachii

Internal oblique

Rectus abdominus

Transverse abdominus

Hip flexors

Quadriceps

Abductors

Adductors

THE MUSCLES OF THE FRONT

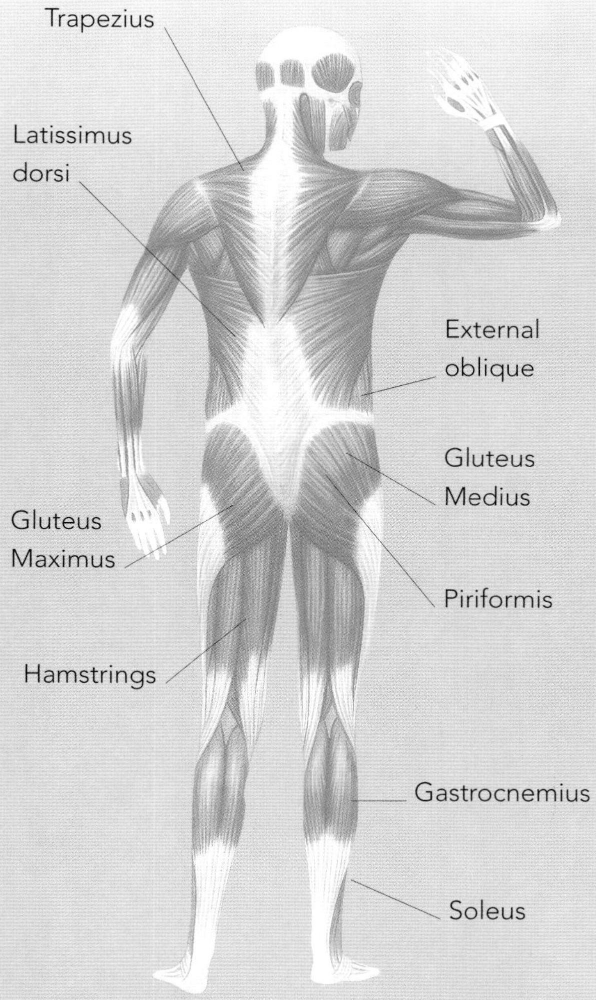

Shoulders, arms, chest and upper back

Strengthening the shoulders, arms, chest and upper back improves functions such as carrying, lifting objects, lifting overhead, pushing and pulling. Sport-specific training of the shoulders and arms benefits sports such as tennis, cricket, volleyball and swimming, as well as the martial arts. Balancing overworked chest muscles with upper back muscles will help to maintain a good posture, prevent injury and assist with rehabilitation after injury.

Abdominals and lower back

The abdominal and lower back muscles are collectively known as the 'core'. 'Core stability' is the ability to control the position and movement of the central portion of the body. Strengthening the abdominal and lower back muscles helps to reduce the risk of injury from bad posture and improves the foundation for all arm and leg movements. In addition, strengthening the abdominals and lower back can prevent and improve lower back pain.

Trapezius

Latissimus dorsi

External oblique

Gluteus Medius

Gluteus Maximus

Piriformis

Hamstrings

Gastrocnemius

Soleus

THE MUSCLES OF THE BACK

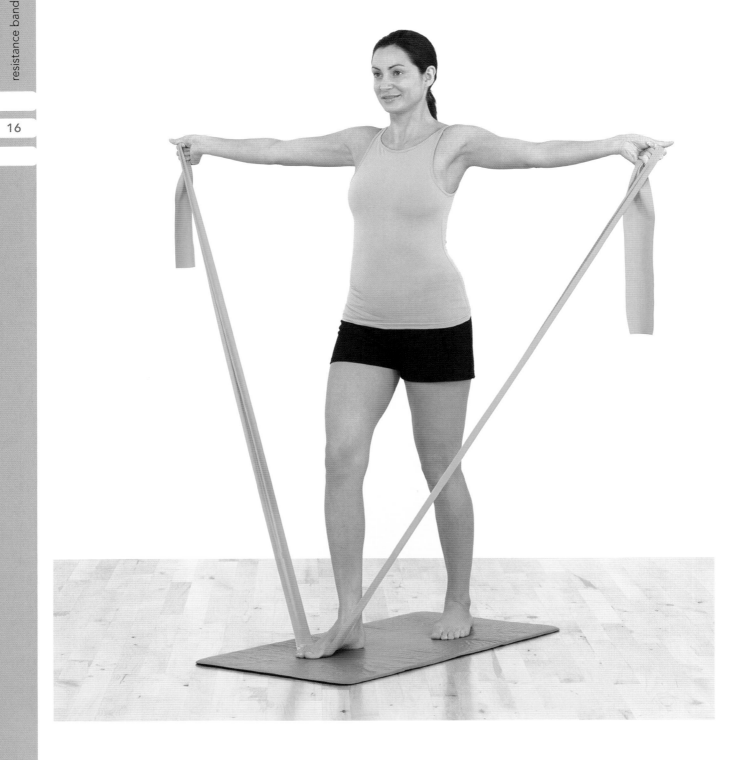

Hips, thighs, lower legs and ankles

The hip and thigh regions are one of the most important areas you can strengthen. Connecting the legs to the trunk, the hips provide a stable base for the 'core'. The hips are fundamental in transferring your centre of gravity during walking and running. The gluteal muscles provide pelvic stability. Weakness of the gluteal muscles is linked to back pain, knee pain, hip pain and repetitive ankle injuries. Also, imbalances of strength and flexibility between your quadriceps and hamstrings can be linked to knee pain.

The lower leg muscles and ankles have important roles with your stability, locomotion and action within the walking and running cycle, known as gait. Improving your lower leg strength can go a long way towards improving your balance and stability, especially when participating in sports that require quick changes of direction, such as football, tennis and basketball.

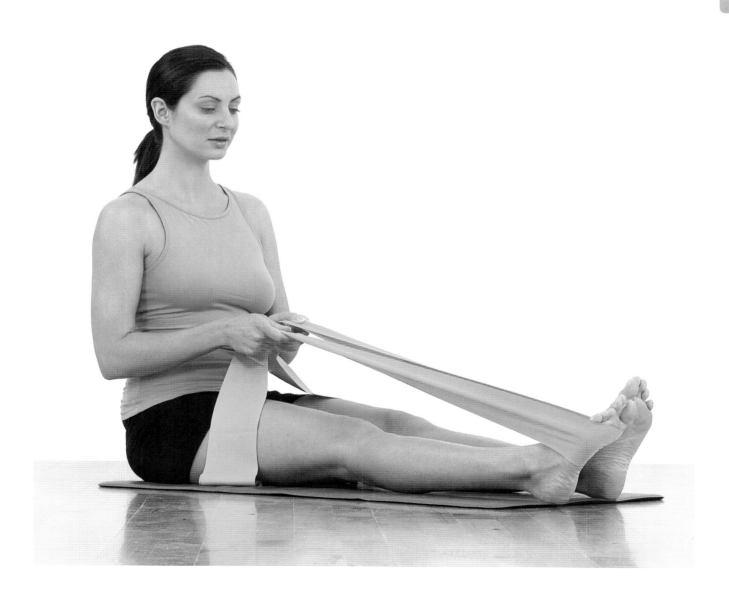

The way our bodies look and respond to different types of exercise is basically determined by our genetics. Other factors include how active you were while growing up, your diet during your childhood and teenage years and your current diet and activity levels.

Often people become disheartened when exercising to lose weight, as they unexpectedly find that their size 'increases'. The reason why is that an increase in muscle bulk within an area with noticeably high body fat can initially cause an increase in that area's overall size. This occurs because anaerobic exercise tends to cause muscles to bulk and increase in size more than aerobic exercise does, and because the body fat has not yet decreased sufficiently and is overlying any area of increased muscle bulk. This can be avoided by exercising correctly for your body type. Body type is not how much fat or muscle your body has. It simply means where on your body it would be evident if weight was being added or lost.

X-types

X-types have the classic hourglass-shaped body, which proportionally tends to add mass to both the upper and lower parts of the body quite easily, while the waist will be more slender. They will also lose mass proportionally from the upper and lower bodies.

Aerobic weight-management resistance band exercises for both upper and lower bodies will benefit the X-type. As they slim down, the exercise can turn more anaerobic.

Y-types

Y-types are bigger on the top half of their body, with a tendency to bulk up from the waist up. Y-types carry weight and mass in their upper back and chest, and their arms are usually large as well.

To reduce the size of the upper part of your body, use an aerobic exercise weight-management plan on

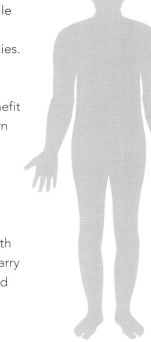

X   Y

body types

your upper body, with a low intensity of resistance band and high repetitions. Y-types will benefit from moderate to high intensity anaerobic resistance band exercises to the lower half of the body.

If you are overweight, reduce the resistance on the upper body, because fat will be pushed outwards as muscle is built.

I-types

I-types carry the same proportion of weight on the upper body as on the lower, are not tapered in their midsection, and do not have many curves.

Provided I-types are not overweight, they can perform both anaerobic and aerobic resistance band exercises. If you are overweight, however, use predominantly aerobic weight-management resistance band exercises.

A-types

A-types are the classic pear shape. Their upper bodies may not be small, yet they are still considerably smaller than their lower half. A-types tend to put on weight or mass in their thighs, hips, behind the knees and even in the calves and ankles.

A-types should use a low-intensity weight-management resistance band exercises at high repetitions for the lower body. You can use anaerobic resistance band exercises of moderate to high resistance at low repetitions for your upper body. If you are overweight, resistance should not be too high for the upper body, because fat will be pushed outwards as muscle is built.

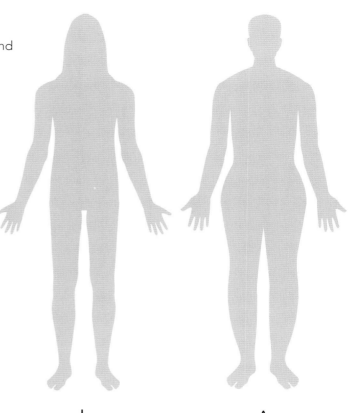

I A

AEROBIC AND ANAEROBIC EXERCISE

Aerobic exercise, such as gentle jogging, is replicated by moderate to low levels of resistance band intensity with high repetitions, maintaining an increased heart rate, but not entering into the anaerobic zone. The aerobic exercise zone is also known as the weight management zone. Anaerobic exercise uses muscles in a brief, high intensity activity where oxygen requirements cannot meet the demand of the activity, increasing the breathing and heart rate very quickly, for example when you are sprinting. A high tension resistance band enabling only low repetitions before fatigue will add to muscle bulk.

To ensure you get the maximum benefit from resistance band exercises, and indeed any exercise, check your heart rate during your fitness session. The number of heartbeats per minute is one of the easiest measures to take, and as you become fitter you will be able to increase your heart rate without straining your heart.

Your target heart rate (THR) is the recommended number of heartbeats per minute for your age and fitness level while exercising. It is derived as a percentage of your maximum heart rate. It is important to remain within the target heart zone to ensure you are exercising with the correct intensity. If you are exercising above your THR, you are exercising too vigorously; below your THR, and you are not exercising with enough vigour.

To take your own pulse, place your two forefingers on your carotid arteries, found either side of your neck, just below the angle of the jaw, between the neck muscle and windpipe. Do not use your thumb because it has a pulse of its own.

Time your heartbeat for 15 seconds. Multiply the number of beats over 15 seconds by four. This will give you your beats per minute.

ZONE LIMIT

Zone	Target heart rate %	ratio of calories burnt (fat/other calories)	Benefit
Warm-up	50–60	85/15	Warm-up and warm-down zones. Decreases body fat, blood pressure and cholesterol.
Weight management	60–70	85/15	As above, but burns more total calories.
Aerobic	70–80	50/50	Improves your cardiovascular and respiratory system, and increases the size and strength of your heart. Builds more 'slow twitch' muscle fibres.
Anaerobic	80–90	15/85	High-intensity zone, burning more calories, improving the cardiorespiratory system and increasing endurance. Builds more 'fast twitch' muscle fibres.

target heart rate

Example
20 beats in 15 seconds = 80 beats per minute

Your maximum heart rate is your age subtracted from 220 for men, and your age subtracted from 226 for women. This number, your maximum heart rate of beats per minute, should not be exceeded during any physical activity.

Example
A 40-year-old man has a maximum heart rate of 180 beats per minute (220 – 40 = 180).

From this, you can then work out the upper and lower limits for your heart rate in the different zones. Simply multiply your maximum heart rate by the upper and lower target heart rates listed in the table opposite.

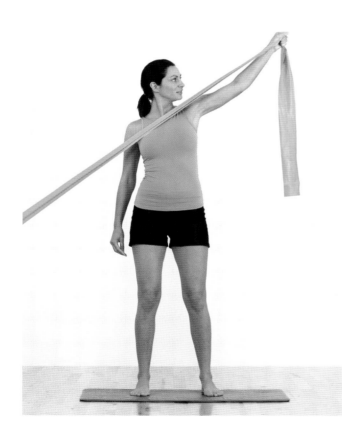

HEART RATE CALCULATIONS

Maximum heart rate for women = 226 - age

Maximum heart rate for men = 220 - age

Upper target heart rate =
(Maximum heart rate) x (upper % of zone)

Lower target heart rate =
(Maximum heart rate) x (lower % of zone)

Example
For a 28-year-old woman who wishes to exercise in the aerobic zone:

Maximum heart rate: 226 – 28 = 198

Upper heart rate: 198 x 0.8 = 158

Lower heart rate: 198 x 0.7 = 139

Thus, a 28-year-old woman exercising in the aerobic zone would maintain their target heart rate between 139 and 158 beats per minute.

To get the pulse count range, simply divide by 4, giving 35 to 39 beats over 15 seconds.

Think of a time in the past when you had a peak moment when you felt good, fit, strong and able, energized and excited – it could be a sporting moment, or even after being able to climb a steep flight of stairs or a challenging hill. Please take a moment, now, and reflect on that time and in your mind relive it. Where were you, what were you doing? Feel as many of the sensory elements of that time as you can recall and bring it to life again – recreate that time as if you were there now and feel alive again.

Now project your thoughts forwards in time, to your reason for exercising with resistance bands and to your desired state. Notice the increased fitness, strength and mobility you can gain. See yourself in that moment, and the benefits you have gained – energy to tackle stairs with ease, improved balance, more vigour to play with your children, greater potential in your sport, or whatever is the desired outcome of these exercises. Notice, too, the improvements to your lifestyle, such as the reduction in stress and the joy that brings you, and hear people telling you how good you look, and asking you how you achieved it.

Motivation is a force that makes us 'do', turning desires and goals into action. There are two types of motivation, positive and negative. Positive motivation comes from a natural response to desire. What do you desire from exercise? Is it the way it makes you look and feel, or could it be the increased strength and stability it will give you during your next skiing holiday, for example? You want to exercise because of the desired outcome.

Negative motivation is derived, in this context, from the result of not exercising. For example, 'I will put on weight if I do not exercise'; 'I must exercise tonight, because if I miss any more sessions I will never

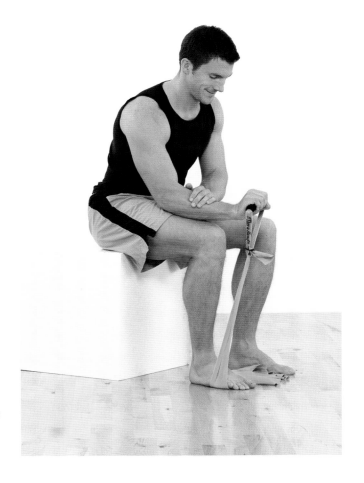

motivation

become fitter', etc. Eventually, negative motivation creates stress. This can cause people to stop exercising, because of the mind's resistance to these negative thoughts.

A way to identify negative motivation is to notice any time you use words like 'should', 'must', 'have to', 'ought to' and 'got to'. Once you have noticed yourself using these words, change them to positive ones like 'want to', 'feel like', 'would like to', etc. It creates less internal resistance from your mind.

Find the positive good in the reasons for exercising correctly and consistently. Notice any negative motivation and transform it into positive, allowing your desire for that positive good to be your primary motivation.

By reading this book you will understand the basic fundamentals of exercise – warming-up, stretching, warming-down, etc – and learn that exercising within your chosen zones will assist you in attaining your desired outcome. Results come through consistency and this is why you will want to set time aside during your week to exercise. Remember that any time you say, 'I should', you can change this to, 'I want to', and 'I must' can become, 'I will'. In doing so, you will notice an elevation of the stress involved and enjoy being empowered to motivate yourself towards your desired result.

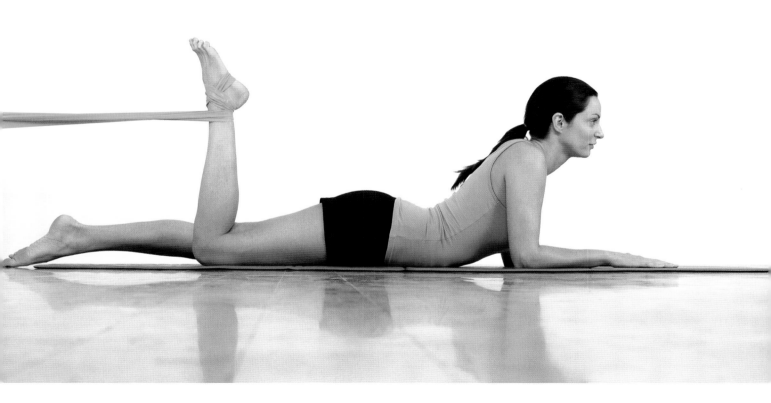

When reading and looking at an exercise or stretch, visualize yourself doing the resistance band exercise before you physically do it. There are several reasons for visualizing, and one of them is to enable you to develop your own set of exercises in time to come. As mentioned earlier, the possibilities for the use of resistance bands in exercise and sport development are limited only by your imagination. This visualization technique will enable you to practise the exercise correctly, so you will maximize the benefit from the exercises and reduce the likelihood of improper resistance band technique and resulting injury.

All top sports people visualize before executing the technique for real. Top golfers, for example, never take a swing, either in practice or in a tournament, without having first visualized the stroke, and when visualizing, they hit the shot perfectly, every time. When you visualize any form of exercise, ensure your technique is perfect.

The reason for this is that when we visualize, picturing with feeling and all our senses active in this visualization, our brain sends minute signals to the muscles involved in the action we are 'seeing'. The neurological pathways are being made, even though we are not actually doing the exercise. A great example many of us have experienced is when we are dreaming. Our body may twitch and seem to move involuntarily in reaction to what we are dreaming. The brain's signals are as if the event were real, and for the muscles it is real, there is no difference.

There is an important link between visualization and motivation. Using negative motivation, stating what you do not want, creates a visual image of what you do not want. This image draws you further towards what you do not want to happen. An example of this negative draw is: 'I do not want to lose my balance.'

Did you think of losing your balance, even though you were trying not to? Using positive motivation leads us towards what we want, our desired outcome. A positive approach to the previous example would be, 'Maintain my balance.'

By reading the exercise instructions and observing the images of that exercise, picture yourself doing the exercise and doing it perfectly and positively. You should be associated with the visualization. That means seeing everything as if through your eyes with feeling – that is, how the motion of the exercise acts on your muscles. Add sounds and other sensory cues that are associated with the event, such as the noise of the band stretching, even the smell of the band. Correct yourself if you notice that you are using statements such as: 'Don't bend my back.' Correct this to: 'Keep my back straight.' By doing so, and by executing the visualized technique perfectly, you are setting yourself up for success. This will help you with your balance and your posture while using the resistance band. This is your body and you can maximize its control and function. Have the motivation to incorporate visualization into your learning of the exercises. Incorporate this into your chosen sport.

visualization

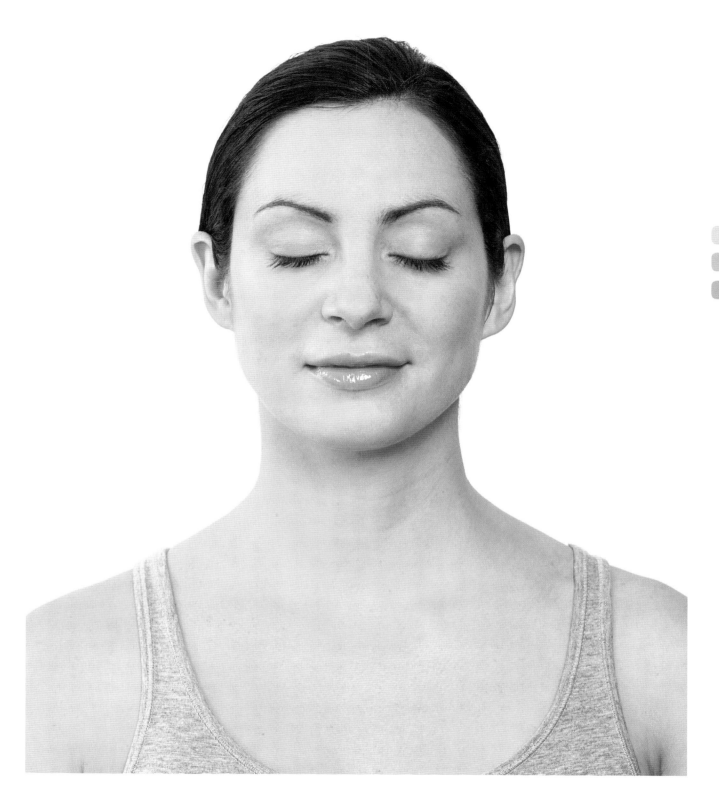

Now that you know all about resistance bands and your body, it is time to bring it together.

A resistance band is wonderfully simple, yet highly effective. Because of its compact nature, you will be able to exercise just about anywhere. You will probably have thought of the many benefits and possibilities the resistance band and its exercises will bring you, especially if you travel often, or are required to be at home for much of the time. The key is consistency.

Having read the section on basic anatomy, you now have an understanding of the different body types and how assorted resistance exercises affect them. So what's next?

• Decide what your goals are if you have not done so already. What is your reason for exercising with resistance bands?

• Look at the body-type section and decide which of the four body types described best matches your own. Be honest with yourself and reassess at any time to ensure you are giving yourself the best type of workout for your needs.

• Work out your maximum heart rate as shown, and practise finding and taking your own pulse. It soon becomes quite easy to calculate your beats per minute. Remember your maximum heart rate, because you will be monitoring your heart's progress as you exercise within the zones, and do not exceed this maximum.

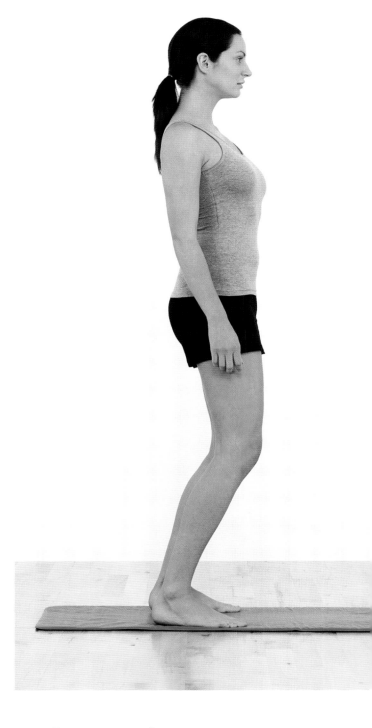

how to use this book

• Knowing why you want to exercise is the key to motivating yourself and being successful. Do practise your awareness and use of motivational words. Notice the words you use to yourself and to others. Are you positively or negatively motivated? Use the simple but truly effective method you have learned for altering and maintaining your motivation.

• The chapters following this introduction will show you how to stretch and exercise with the resistance band, and offer you sample exercise charts. Once you have read through the exercises and the charts you will be able to decide upon the right type of exercises for you and the resistance intensity with which to perform them.

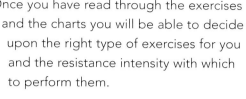

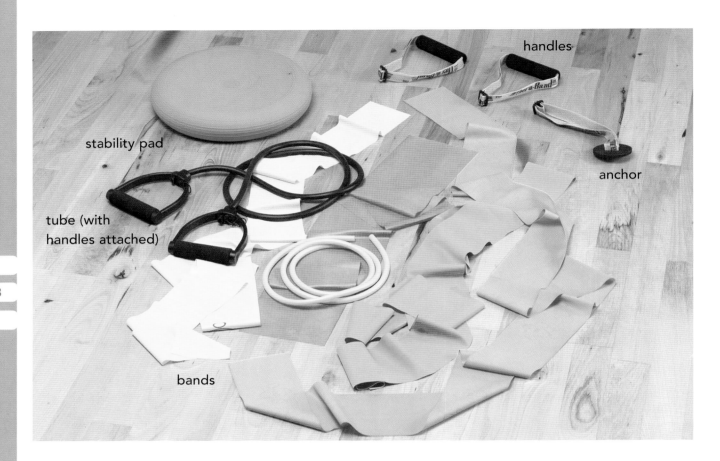

handles

stability pad

tube (with
handles attached)

anchor

bands

Resistance bands, tubes and accessories

There are many elastic band resistance products on the market, most developed from the two basic options of the resistance band and the resistance tube. The two do not differ in principle, concept or mechanics. Choosing between a band and a tube is a matter of personal preference. Bands tend to be favoured as they can be simply wrapped about the hand or body part, without having to be attached to a fixed object. Tubes tend to be preferred for upper body exercises and bands for lower. Tubes and bands are also produced in closed loops and in various dimensions.

Both bands and tubing come in different lengths and many resistance levels. The bands or tubes are colour-coded according to their resistance levels. Generally, both the colour and resistance of the band and tube start light and progress through to darker colours, representing increased resistance.

Products are generally made from Latex, although Latex-free resistance products are available for those with a Latex allergy.

It is important to attach the end of the band securely to prevent injury. There are numerous useful accessories available to enhance your resistance training, such as door anchors and handles. These provide additional safety and comfort when training.

The door anchor is a flat nylon strap with a buckled loop at one end to attach the resistance band or tube and a firm foam pad at the other. Simply position the anchor's flat nylon strap by the door frame with the foam pad positioned on the opposite side of the door frame, then close the door and lock it. This will ensure that the resistance band or tube can be held in position firmly and safely when you apply force to it when exercising.

Safety

- Get approval from your health adviser before undertaking resistance exercises, especially if you have musculoskeletal problems.

- Use Latex-free products if you have a Latex allergy.

- Ensure the band is secured to your chosen anchor point. If using a door as an anchor point, make sure it is securely closed and locked to prevent sudden opening.

- Protect the resistance band from jewellery, sharp objects and fingernails.

- Note that bands degrade if left out in direct sunlight and extremes of temperature.

- Never point a band under tension towards your face.

- Follow the pre- and post-exercise guidelines explained in this book. Ensure you first warm up and then stretch before exercising and warm down when you have completed your workout.

- Maintain correct posture when exercising.

- If you feel pain during an exercise, stop immediately. Reassess to ensure that you are doing the exercise correctly and that you have not skipped your pre-exercise warm-up and stretching phase. Reduce the tension used during that exercise. If pain persists, consult your health professional.

- If your heart rate increases faster and is unusually high during warm-up and/or during exercise, stop exercising. It is an indication that you are tired and your immune system could be fighting off the beginnings of an illness. If symptoms persist, visit your health care professional.

Posture and form

It is important to maintain good posture when exercising. This will reduce the chances of injury and give you maximum benefit from each exercise. The visualization technique will assist you to maintain proper posture and form throughout the exercises.

When standing, have your feet shoulder-width apart, unless otherwise stated, with soft knees (not locked). Keep your lower back and neck in a neutral position, with your shoulders back and down. Make sure you do not twist or arch your back to complete an exercise. Stabilize your torso and improve your core stability by strengthening your abdominal and lower back muscles when exercising. Activate your core muscles by sucking in your stomach while exhaling, and, when you feel your stomach muscles contract, lock them into this contracted position and continue to breathe normally. Activating your core muscles will give you maximum benefit when exercising and improve your results.

The correct motion of the exercise is a combination of your posture and technique or form. When muscles become tired, there is a tendency to 'cheat' by employing different muscle groups to assist, which can lead to injury. Ensure smooth and controlled extensions and contractions during each exercise and maintain your breathing.

BREATHING

Never hold your breath during any part of the exercise, as this can lead to light-headedness or even fainting. Exhale slowly as you apply tension and inhale through the return phase.

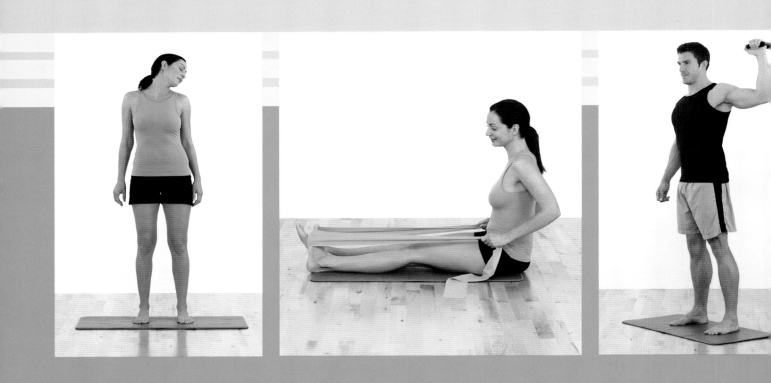

2

warm-up and stretching

In this chapter you will learn why it is essential to warm-up and stretch and to include a proper warm-down after you exercise. The benefits of these will be explained, as well as how these elements will help you towards your desired goal.

The warm-up increases your body temperature and the temperature deep within your muscles. Warming up raises your heart rate gradually, preparing you both physically and mentally for your resistance band exercises to come.

Stretching should only commence after you have warmed up. Stretching will do much more than just increase your flexibility, and in this chapter you will learn why it is so important.

Warming down after exercise is equally important, and you will only receive the full benefits of your exercise when you have cooled down properly.

You will gain maximum benefit from resistance band exercise if you follow the fundamental phases of exercise – warm-up, stretch, exercise and warm-down.

A general warm-up will prepare both your body and mind for exercise. It begins with gentle joint rotation. Start either from your fingers and work your way down, or from your toes and work your way up. These gentle rotations, in both clockwise and anticlockwise directions, facilitate the joints to release synovial fluid, a lubricant that increases the joint's mobility and function when called upon during exercise.

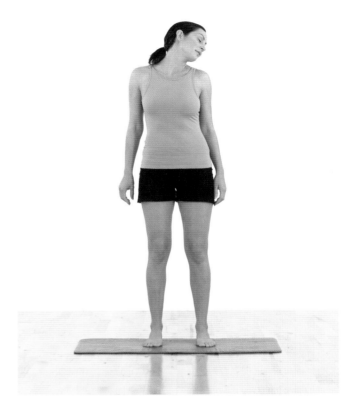

JOINT ROTATION

fingers and knuckles • wrists • elbows • shoulders • neck • trunk/waist • hips • legs • knees • ankles • toes

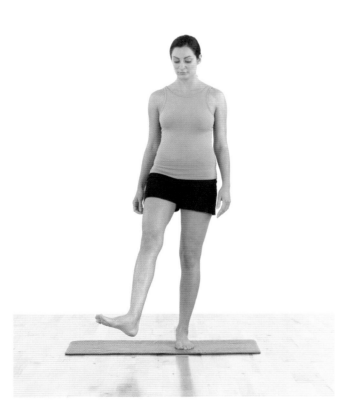

After performing the joint rotations, you should engage in light aerobic activity such as jogging on the spot, light skipping (jump rope), stationary cycling or easy rowing. It should be of sufficient duration and intensity to raise your heart rate to about 50–60% of your maximum heart rate without developing fatigue. It should take between 5 and 15 minutes for your body to feel loose and break into a steady sweat, raising your core body temperature and getting your blood flowing. Increased blood flow in your muscles improves muscle performance and flexibility and reduces the likelihood of injury.

No more than 10 minutes should elapse between completing your warm-up and performing the resistance band exercises.

Once warmed up, begin to stretch. Engage in some slow, relaxed, static stretching, taking between 4 and 7 minutes depending upon your age and flexibility. Start with your back, followed by your upper body and lower body, stretching all your major muscle groups.

Stretching increases your flexibility, which helps to increase your body tone and your ability to avoid injury, and increases your range of motion. Never bounce up and down or stretch until you feel pain. Correct static stretches target the muscle and connecting tissues passively. Stretch until you feel a mild tension, then relax by exhaling a deep breath, then breathe normally as you maintain the stretch. This method enables the muscles to lengthen to their greatest possible extent.

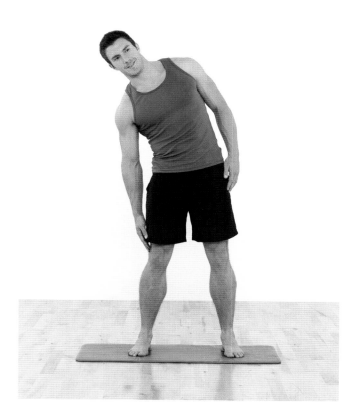

PNF STRETCHING

One of the most effective methods of stretching is called proprioceptive neuromuscular facilitation (PNF). You can facilitate a PNF stretch utilizing the resistance band.

• Take the joint to the end of its range of motion, stretching until you feel a mild tension, then relax with an exhalation of a deep breath. Now breathe normally, maintaining the stretch.

• Utilizing the resistance band, apply mild force (10–20%) muscle pressure against the band in the opposite direction to your stretch for 6 seconds, then relax your resistance, allowing the band's tension to stretch your muscle further to its new lengthened position for another 10–20 seconds. Allow the resistance band to ease the muscle gently into this lengthened position without any input from you, except that of relaxing.

• Again apply 10–20% muscle pressure against the band in the opposite direction to your stretch for 6 seconds, then again relax your resistance, allowing the band's tension to stretch your muscle further to its new lengthened position. Remain in this new position for 10–20 seconds to set your muscle's new length. Repeat this PNF stretching process 3–4 times.

Upper trapezius PNF stretch

Imagine the movement of bringing your left shoulder and your left ear close together by shrugging your left shoulder and tilting your head to the right. Take a moment, now, to visualize this movement, ending with a deep breath and exhaling, releasing any tension the image created, and then relax.

1 Stand with your left foot in the middle of a doubled band. Clasp the ends of the band in your left hand, ensuring there is tension in the band when your left arm is fully extended downwards at your side.

2 Tilt your head to the right and look downwards, using your right hand to hold your head gently in this position.

3 Keeping your left arm straight, shrug your left shoulder upwards, applying mild (10–20%) force on the band. At the same time, use your right hand to resist gently the movement of your head. The rest of your spine remains straight. Hold this position for 6 seconds, breathing naturally throughout.

4 Taking a deep breath, exhale and gently relax both your head and shoulder, allowing the resistance band to release your shoulder downwards, with your right hand maintaining your head tilted towards the right. This will lengthen your upper left trapezius.

5 Breathing normally, hold this position for 10–15 seconds.

6 Repeat the stretch 3–4 times on the left side, then repeat the exercise on the right side.

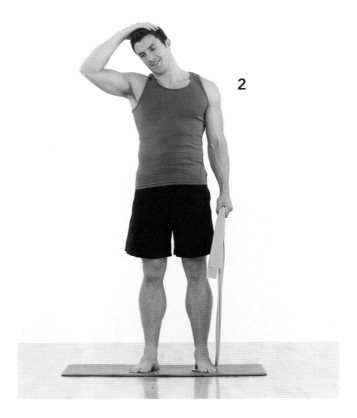

2

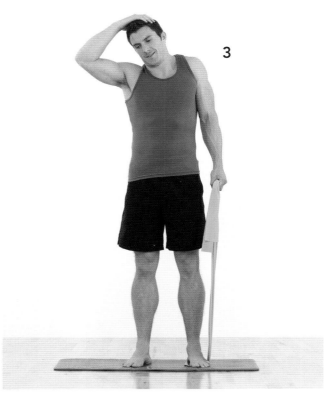

3

Pectoralis major

Overworking the chest area can shorten the pectoralis major muscles, restricting your ability to lift your arms above your head. It also causes forwards or medial rotation of the shoulder, so that when you swing your arms when you walk, your palms face backwards and not to your sides.

1 Secure a doubled resistance band at shoulder height to a fixed object, such as a locked door, using a resistance band anchor.

2 Clasping the band in your left hand, stand with your back to the anchor point and your left elbow and shoulder both at 90-degree angles, as if taking an oath. The band's tension should be enough to stretch the front part of your shoulder gently.

3 Maintaining your elbow position, gently rotate your shoulder inwards with 10–20% force against the resistance band. Hold this static position, breathing normally throughout, for 6 seconds.

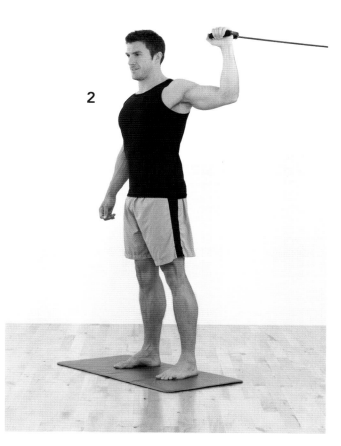

35

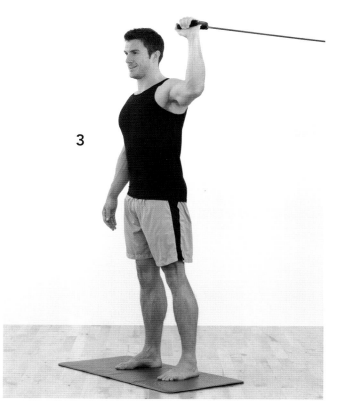

4 Take a deep breath, then relax as you exhale slowly. Allow the band to return your shoulder to just beyond your start position. Notice the reduction in tension within the pectoralis major muscle as you exhale and relax, increasing the muscle's length.

5 Breathing normally, hold this position for 10–15 seconds.

6 Repeat the stretch 3–4 times, then repeat the exercise on the right side.

Quadriceps

The quadriceps are the group of four muscles located to the front of each thigh. Ensuring that these muscles are flexible can assist the correct movement of your knees when walking or running and can help relieve lower back pain.

1 Lie on your front with the resistance band looped around your right shin or foot and your right knee bent to around a 90-degree angle.

2 With the resistance band stretching from your foot passing over your right shoulder, hold the ends of the band in both hands with your arms stretched out in front of you. Ensure you are in a stable and comfortable position on the floor. Maintain enough tension in the resistance band so that it stretches your quadriceps until you feel a mild tension.

3 Start to apply 10–20% of your quadriceps' strength, opposing the pull of the resistance band by initiating the straightening of your right knee. Your lower leg will move slightly away from your body as the resistance band absorbs your force, then remain in a static position, with the force of the band equal to that of your quadriceps. Hold this position for 6 seconds, breathing naturally throughout.

4 Taking a deep breath, exhale and gently relax the quadriceps, allowing the resistance band to return your knee to the start position. Notice your knee has bent a little further, which is normal as the quadriceps have lengthened with the stretch. Breathing normally, hold this position for 10–20 seconds.

5 Repeat the stretch 3–4 times, then repeat the exercise on the left side.

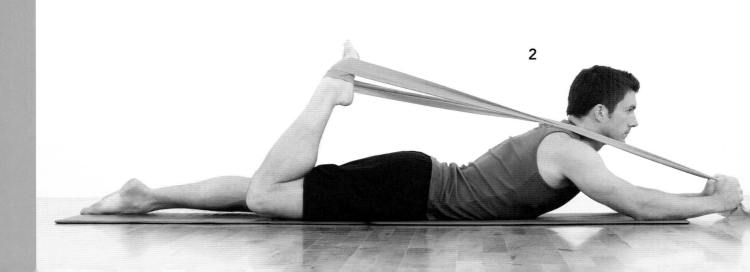

2

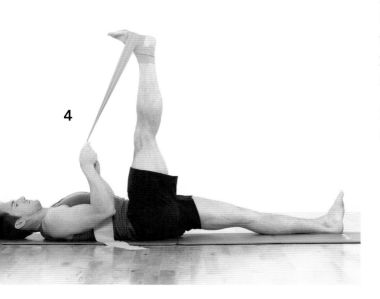

Hamstrings

The hamstrings are the group of three muscles located at the rear of each thigh. Ensuring these powerful muscles are flexible can assist in preventing knee pain and can help relieve lower back pain.

1 Lie on your back with both legs flat and the resistance band looped under your right foot. Hold the ends of the band in both hands.

2 Keeping your leg straight, use the band to lift your right leg upwards, until you feel a mild tension in your hamstrings.

3 Push the right leg downwards towards the floor with 10–20% force against the resistance band, keeping your knee straight. You will probably need to pull with your hands to increase the amount of force being applied by the band to equal the downward movement of your leg. Hold this position for 6 seconds, breathing normally.

4 With a deep breath, exhale and relax your hamstrings, allowing the resistance band to pull your leg gently back towards and beyond your extended starting position. Notice that your hamstrings will have lengthened. Ensure that your back remains flat on the floor and you are not lifting your hips or your left leg off the floor. Hold this relaxed stretched position for 10–20 seconds.

5 Repeat the stretch 3–4 times, then repeat the exercise on the left side.

THINK POSITIVELY

Remember your desired outcome and why it is important to stretch before you exercise. Alter any negative motivational thoughts, such as 'I should…', to positive motivational words, such as 'I want…'.

Hip flexor

Imagine kneeling on your left knee, with your right foot on the floor in front of you, right knee bent to no more than 90 degrees, in the classic 'will you marry me' proposal position. Make sure your shoulders and hips are square and facing forwards. This is the basic position for this stretch.

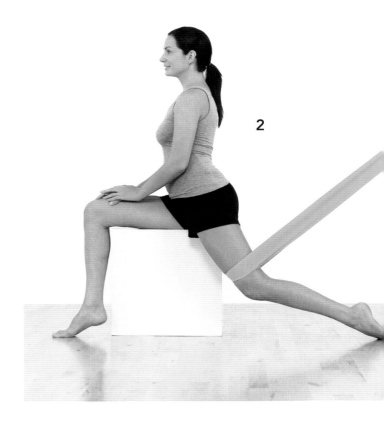

1 Secure a doubled resistance band at waist height to a solid object, such as a locked door, using a resistance band anchor.

2 Loop the band around your left thigh, just above your knee. Side-sit on a solid chair with your back to the band's attachment point. Your right buttock and thigh should be supported on the chair, the right knee bent to 90 degrees and your right foot on the floor. Make sure your hips and pelvis are square and your back is straight. Assume the proposal position, with your left hip gently extended behind, left knee slightly bent. Allow the resistance band to apply mild tension to your hip and thigh muscles, adjusting your distance from the anchor point to apply sufficient tension.

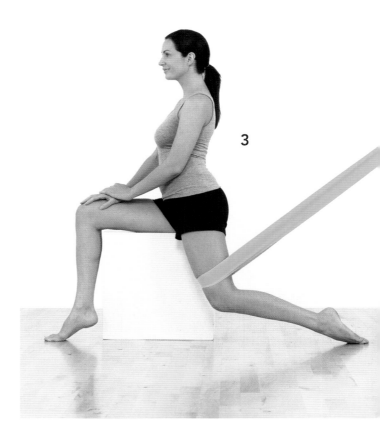

3 Gently flex your left hip forwards against the band's tension, 10–20% force, for 6 seconds, breathing normally. With a deep breath, exhale and relax your hip, allowing the resistance band to gently extend your hip backwards beyond your starting position. Hold this relaxed stretched position for 10–20 seconds.

4 Repeat the stretch 3–4 times, then repeat the exercise on the other side.

Gastrocnemius and soleus

The gastrocnemius and soleus muscles are located at the rear of the lower leg. Commonly known as the calf muscles, they are fundamental for running and jumping. Constant wearing of high-heeled shoes causes these muscles to shorten, which can affect posture negatively. The two muscles of the calf are stretched in similar ways except that the knee is slightly bent when stretching the soleus, whereas the gastrocnemius stretch requires your leg to be straight.

1 Sitting on the floor, with legs straight, loop the resistance band under the ball of your left foot.

2 Holding the ends of the band in both hands, stretch the band, pulling your foot backwards until you feel mild tension in your calf muscles. Gently push the foot forwards using 10–20% force for 6 seconds, breathing normally. You might need to pull on the band to adjust the tension at this point, to balance the force exerted by your foot.

3 Exhale deeply as you relax your calf muscles, allowing the band to pull your foot backwards beyond your starting position, again until you feel mild tension. Hold this relaxed position for 10–15 seconds while breathing normally.

4 Repeat the stretch 3–4 times, then repeat the exercise on the right side.

STRETCHING

Stretching increases your flexibility, which helps to increase your body tone and your ability to avoid injury and also increases your range of motion. Never bounce up and down or stretch until you feel pain.

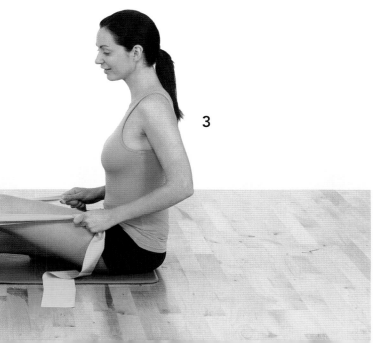

3

Piriformis

The piriformis muscles are located in the buttocks. A common problem that can be associated with tight piriformis muscles is sciatic pain, which can be reduced by stretching and lengthening these muscles.

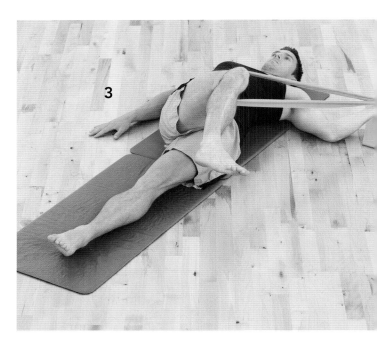

1 Lie flat on your back with both legs extended. Keeping your left leg flat on the floor, lift and bend your right leg and lay it across your left knee. Loop the resistance band over your right thigh, just above your knee, and clasp the ends of the band in your left hand. Extend your right arm out to the side to give you extra stability, making sure your back remains in contact with the floor.

2 Gently pull the band so that your right leg crosses further over your left knee until you feel mild tension in the right piriformis.

3 Gently pull your right thigh back towards your right side, applying 10–20% force with your right knee against the band. Breathing normally, hold the position for 6 seconds, with the force of the band equal to that of your thigh.

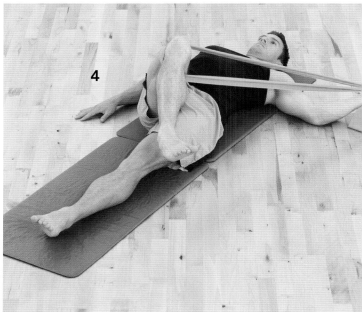

4 Exhale and relax your piriformis, letting the resistance band pull your right leg back to beyond the starting position until mild tension is felt. Remain relaxed by breathing normally. Maintain this position for 10–20 seconds.

5 Repeat the stretch 3–4 times, then repeat the exercise on the left side.

BREATHING

Never hold your breath when stretching or exercising. Exhaling after a deep breath enables you to release muscle tension in your body. This enables the muscles to relax more and therefore increases their length.

Latissimus dorsi and internal obliques

The latissimus dorsi and internal oblique muscles are heavily utilized in sports such as golf, all throwing sports, gymnastics, swimming and rowing. This great stretch will assist you in increasing both your mobility and your range of movement.

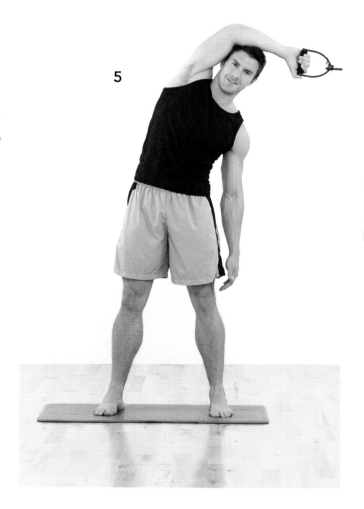

5

1 Securely attach the resistance band at a high level, such as at the top of a locked door, using a resistance band anchor. Stand with your left side towards the anchor point. Clasp the end of the resistance band in your right hand, with your arm raised high above your shoulder, thumb inwards.

2 Move sideways away from the anchor point until the resistance band is taut. Stand with your feet close together, ensuring that you do not lean either forwards or backwards.

3 Keeping your right arm raised and your left foot stationary, take a side step to the right, away from the anchor point.

4 Lean your trunk towards the anchor point, allowing the resistance band to draw a mild stretch to your latissimus dorsi and internal oblique muscles on the right side.

5 Lean your trunk towards the right and gently apply 10–20% force, pulling against the resistance band. Breathing normally, hold this position for 6 seconds.

6 Exhale and relax your torso, letting the resistance band stretch you beyond your starting position until mild tension is felt. Remain relaxed by breathing normally. Maintain this position for 10–20 seconds.

7 Repeat the stretch 3–4 times, then repeat the exercise on the right side.

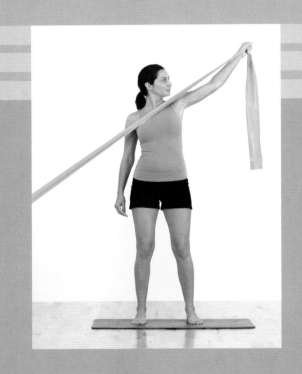
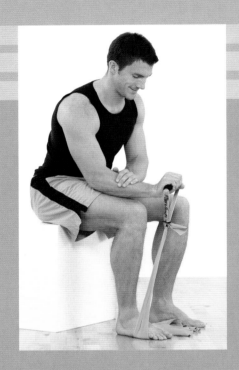
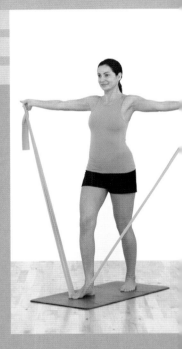

3

shoulder and arm exercises

Strengthening the shoulders and arms improves functions such as carrying, lifting overhead and pushing, and may prevent injury. The unique benefits of training with resistance bands allow you to move more freely and achieve a greater range of motion, as opposed to machines, which control where you start and stop. Being able to create resistance from any direction – high overhead, below from floor level or to the side – resistance bands allow you to imitate movements that you do in real life and exercise muscles that machines miss. This benefits sport-specific training of the shoulders and arms, useful for many sports such as tennis, cricket and volleyball, and the martial arts.

Over shoulder press

This exercise targets your shoulders, helping to improve your ability to lift or push. It also increases your strength when reaching overhead.

1 Stand with the middle of the band under your right foot. If using handles, ensure they are securely attached to the ends of the resistance band, though handles are not essential. Keep your feet shoulder-width apart, but with the left foot slightly in front, and your knees slightly bent (known as soft knees). Hold the ends of the band at shoulder level.

2 Lift your hands above your head, straightening your elbows. Hold this position for a count of one, then return your hands to shoulder height slowly and with control.

3 Reverse your position to work the left side.

Variation
To initiate your core stability, perform the exercise while standing on one leg, and for an additional challenge place a foam- or air-filled stability pad under that foot. Alternate the leg you stand on during core stability, completing half your repetitions on each leg.

CAUTION

If you experience shoulder pain during this exercise, stop and reassess your technique and the resistance of the band. Use a band with less resistance. If pain persists, consult your health professional.

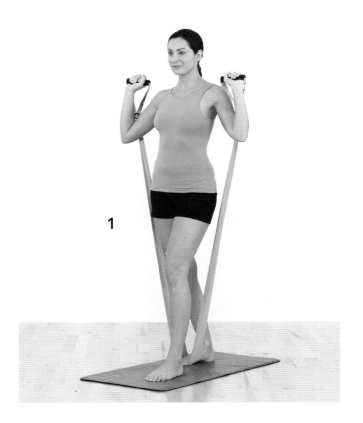

1

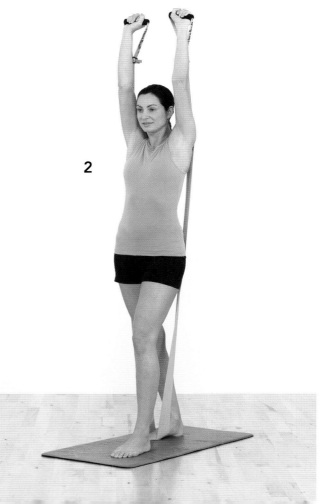

2

Shoulder lateral raise

This is an intensive exercise for your shoulders. It can also help to improve your reach out to the sides, a movement that is essential in many sports.

1 Stand with the middle of the band under your right foot. Holding one end of the band in each hand, start with both arms extended down by your sides.

2 Keeping your thumbs upwards, lift both arms outwards and upwards slowly and with control, keeping your elbows straight. Stop for a count of one at shoulder level, then return your arms back to the start position.

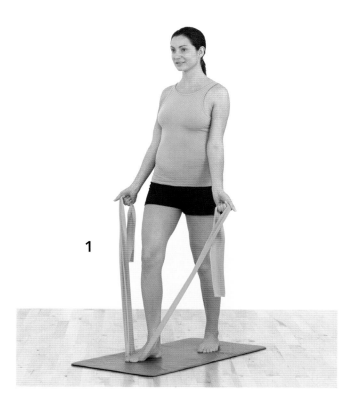

1

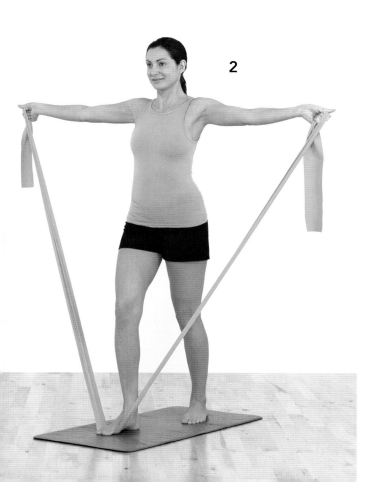

2

Variations

Take your arms completely over your head, again keeping your thumbs upwards. To work your core stability, perform the exercise standing on one leg, and for an additional challenge place a foam- or air-filled stability pad under that foot. Alternate the leg you stand on during core stability, completing half your repetitions on each leg.

TIP

Avoid shrugging your shoulders by keeping your shoulder blades down; maintain a straight back and remember to breathe normally throughout the exercise. Exhale slowly as you apply tension and inhale through the return phase. It is important to control your technique with a smooth controlled motion. There is no rush.

Shoulder diagonal flexion

This exercise targets the shoulders, but it also works other muscles, especially when you work your core stability at the same time.

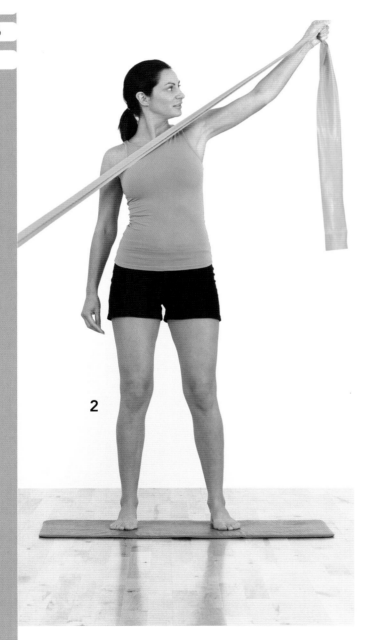

2

1 Use a resistance band anchor to secure the resistance band at low level, such as the bottom of a locked door. Stand with your right side to the anchor point, with your feet shoulder-width apart and knees slightly bent.

2 Clasp the end of the band with your left hand, keeping the elbow straight. Starting with your left hand at your right hip, pull the band upwards and outwards away from your body and across your torso, ending with your left arm extended high above your head. Follow your hand with your eyes to help you control the movement, and maintain a straight back and tight abdominals at all times. Hold this position for a count of one. The exercise is only half complete – maintain your concentration.

3 Return your arm slowly and with control to the start position.

4 Reverse your position to work the right side.

Shoulder diagonal extension

Strengthening the shoulders will help towards preventing shoulder injuries and assist rehabilitation, helping you achieve your potential.

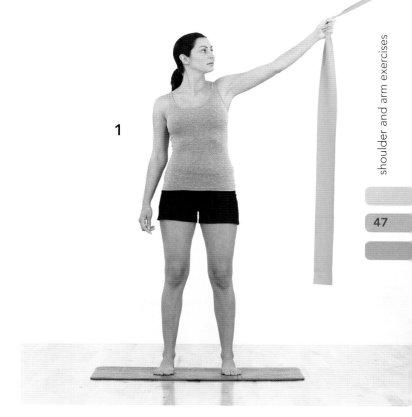

CAUTION

If the hand holding the resistance band begins to sweat, stop momentarily and dry your hand and the band using a towel. Letting go of a fully tensioned band can be dangerous.

1 Using a resistance band anchor, attach the resistance band securely at high level, such as the top of a locked door. Stand with your left side facing the anchor point, with your feet shoulder-width apart and knees slightly bent.

2 Clasp the end of the band with your left hand, keeping the elbow straight, starting with the left hand high above your head. Pull the band downwards and across your torso, ending with your left hand at the right hip. Follow your hand with your eyes to help you control the movement, and maintain a straight back and tight abdominals at all times. Hold this position for a count of one. The exercise is only half complete – maintain your concentration.

3 Return your arm slowly and with control to the start position.

4 Reverse your position to work the right side.

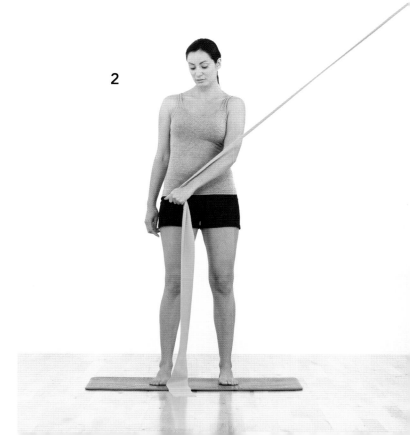

Shoulder rotations

These exercises are particularly good for anyone who takes part in racket sports or plays golf.

Shoulder Internal Rotation

1 Using a resistance band anchor, attach the resistance band securely to a locked door at elbow level. If using a handle, make sure it is securely attached to the end of the resistance band. Place a rolled towel under your right arm – although this is not essential, it can assist you in controlling the motion of the exercise.

2 Stand with your right side facing the anchor point, with your feet shoulder-width apart and knees slightly bent. Clasp the end of the band with your right hand, keeping your right elbow by your side and bent at 90 degrees so that your forearm is parallel to the floor. Ensure the band is taut, and maintain a straight back and tight abdominals at all times.

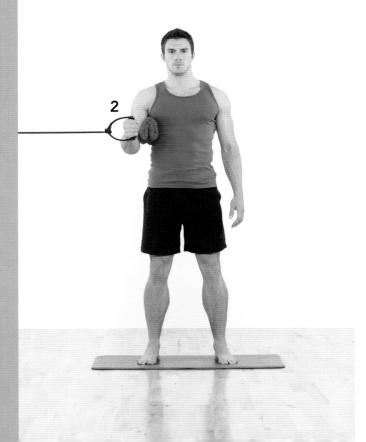

3 Slowly pivot your forearm towards your torso, away from the anchor point, without extending your elbow or your wrist to complete the motion. Hold this position for a count of one, then return to the start position slowly and with control. Remember to exhale slowly as you apply tension and inhale through the return phase – never hold your breath.

4 Reverse your position to work the left side.

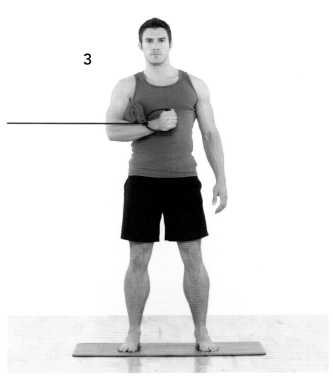

Shoulder External Rotation

To perform the external rotation, start the exercise in the same position as the internal rotation with your right side facing the anchor point. However, place the rolled towel under your left arm and clasp the end of the band with your left hand. Keep your left elbow by your side and bent at 90 degrees so that your forearm is parallel to the floor. Slowly pivot your forearm away from your torso and away from the anchor point, without extending your elbow or your wrist to complete the motion. Hold this position for a count of one, then return to the start position slowly and with control. Reverse your position to work the right side.

Triceps pull-down

The triceps are located at the rear of our upper arms. This simple and effective exercise ensures they're not neglected.

1 Using a resistance band anchor, attach the resistance band securely at high level, such as the top of a locked door. Stand facing the anchor point. Position your feet one slightly in front of the other for stability, and with knees slightly bent.

2 Clasp one end of the resistance band in each hand, with your upper arms fixed by your sides and your elbows bent at 45 degrees. Make sure the resistance band is taut; if not, move a little further away from the anchor point.

3 Straighten your elbows, concentrating on maintaining their position by your sides without moving your shoulders. When your elbows are at full extension with the palms of your hands facing backwards, hold this position for a count of one, then return your elbows to the start position slowly and with control.

2

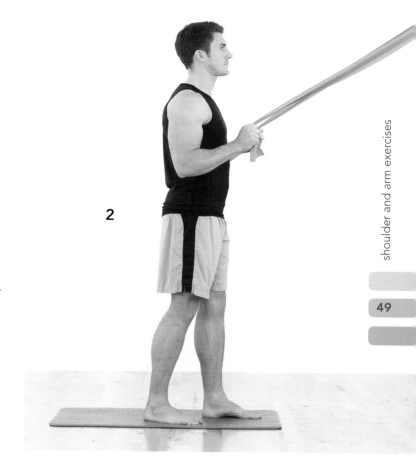

3

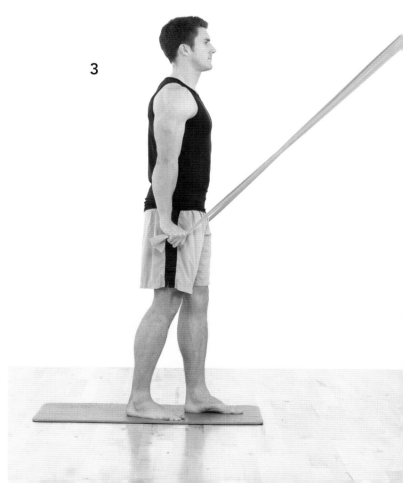

Biceps curl

This straightforward exercise is very effective at improving your upper arm strength.

1 Stand with your right foot in the middle of your band and your knees slightly bent.

2 Clasp one end of the resistance band in your right hand. If using a handle, ensure it is securely attached to the end of the resistance band. With your right arm by your side and your elbow straight, the resistance band should be taut; if the band is not taut, either adjust your grip further down the band's length or, if using a handle, shorten the band's length. Begin with your right palm forwards and your arms by your sides, elbows straight. Activate your core muscles and maintain their tension throughout the exercise.

TIP

Ensure that your back remains straight throughout the exercise and do not use other muscles to complete the full range of motion. If you are unable to maintain a controlled motion in both the flexion and extension of your elbow, use a band with less resistance.

3 Keeping your upper right arm fixed at your side the whole time, bend your right elbow, bringing your hand slowly up towards your chest. Pause for a count of one, then release your hands to the start position slowly and with control.

4 Reverse your position to work the left side.

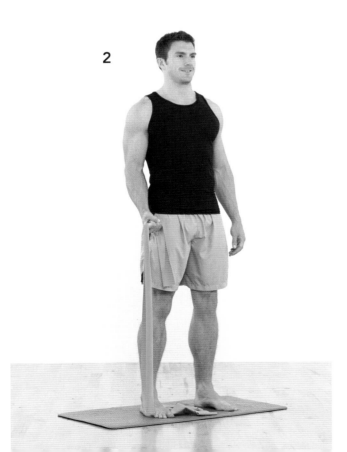

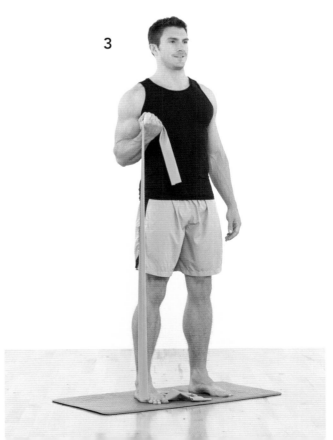

Wrist curl

These wrist curl exercises benefit all racket sports and can help to reduce tennis and golfer's elbow.

1 Sit comfortably on a chair. Secure the length of the resistance band under your left foot and hold the end in your left hand. If using a handle, ensure it is securely attached to the end of the resistance band.

2 Bend your left elbow and stabilize your forearm on your left thigh, with your palm turned upwards and your wrist fully extended. Make sure the resistance band is taut.

3 Now flex your wrist slowly upwards, ensuring that you do not use your elbow to complete the exercise. Hold this position for a count of one, then return to the start position smoothly and with control.

4 Reverse your position to work the right wrist.

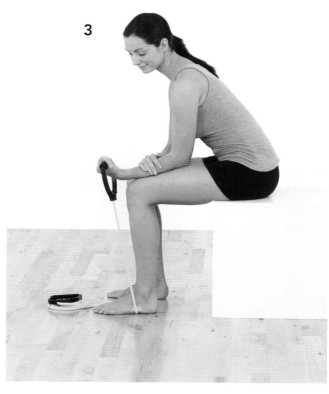

3

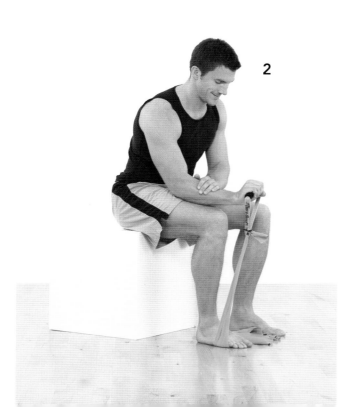

2

Reverse wrist curl

1 Sit comfortably in a chair. Secure the length of the resistance band under your right foot and hold the end in your right hand. If using a handle, ensure it is securely attached to the end of the resistance band.

2 Bend your right elbow and stabilize your forearm on your right thigh, with your palm turned downwards and your wrist fully flexed. Make sure the resistance band is taut.

3 Now slowly straighten your wrist, ensuring that you do not use your elbow to complete the exercise. Hold this position for a count of one, then return to the start position smoothly and with control.

4 Reverse your position to work the right wrist.

Wrist forearm pronation

This exercise strengthens
the motion that rotates your
wrists when you turn your
palms downwards.

1 Using a resistance band anchor, secure one end of
the resistance band to be level with your hips when
you are seated. Secure the other end of the band
using a 'sports handle' accessory or the handle of a
tennis racket or squash racket. Sit on a chair with your
left side to the anchor point and hold the handle in
your left hand.

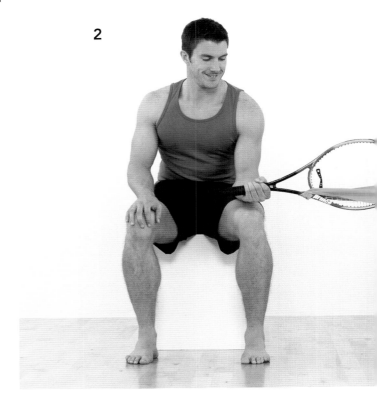

2

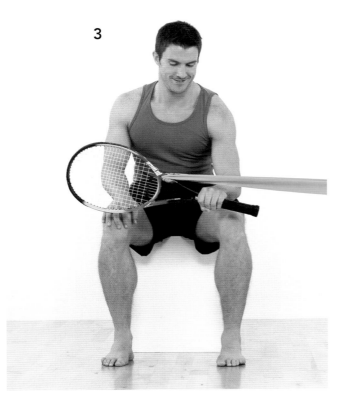

3

2 Bend your left elbow and stabilize your forearm
on your left thigh, with your palm turned upwards,
ensuring the resistance band is taut.

3 Now rotate your hand slowly to the right. Hold
this position for a count of one, then return to the
start position smoothly and with control.

4 Reverse your position to work the right side.

TIP

Keep your elbow in this fixed position, ensuring you
do not use your elbow to complete the exercise.

Wrist forearm supination

This is the reverse of the previous exercise, strengthening the motion that rotates your wrists when you turn your palms upwards.

1 Using a resistance band anchor, secure one end of the resistance band to be level with your hips when you are seated. Secure the other end of the band using a 'sports handle' accessory or the handle of a tennis racket or squash racket. Sit on a chair with your left side square on to the anchor point and hold the handle in your right hand.

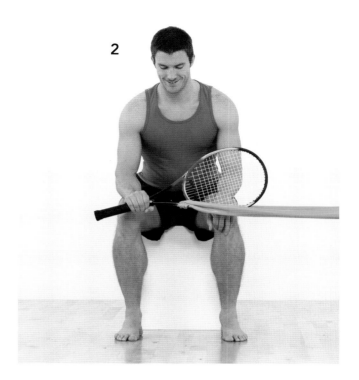

2 Bend your right elbow and stabilize your forearm on your right thigh, with your palm turned downwards, ensuring the resistance band is taut.

3 Now rotate your hand slowly to the right. Hold this position for a count of one, then return to the start position smoothly and with control.

4 Reverse your position to work the right side.

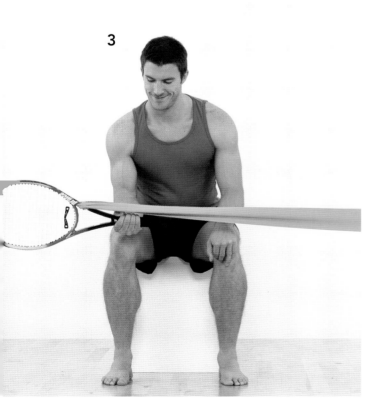

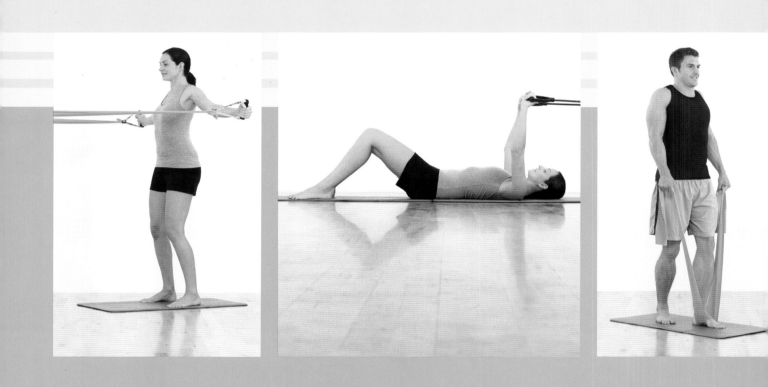

4

chest and upper back exercises

Working with a resistance band, you can reproduce exercises for the chest and upper back performed with traditional strengthening equipment and machines. Strengthening your chest and upper back can assist in the prevention and rehabilitation of shoulder and neck injuries. Improvements in functions such as pushing and pulling and carrying objects are attainable with the resistance band equipment and exercises. Sports-specific training of the chest and upper back muscles, involving movements that you do in real life, benefit sporting activities such as tennis, cricket, volleyball, swimming and the martial arts.

Standing bench press

Resistance bands are extremely versatile – this exercise enables you to bench press without the need for excessive equipment and heavy weights.

1 Using a resistance band anchor, attach the resistance band securely to a locked door above shoulder level. If using handles, make sure they are securely attached to the ends of the resistance band.

2 Stand with your back towards the anchor point. Keep your feet shoulder-width apart, but with one foot slightly in front of the other, and knees slightly bent. Start the exercise holding the ends of the resistance band at around shoulder level with elbows bent and palms downwards, ensuring the band is taut.

3 Keeping your back and neck straight, extend your arms, pushing the resistance band forwards until your arms are straight out in front of you, without shrugging your shoulders. Make sure your shoulders remain square and both arms are extending at the same rate. Hold this position for a count of one, then return to the start position slowly and with control.

Variations
To work your core stability, perform the exercise standing on one leg, and for an additional challenge place a foam- or air-filled stability pad under your foot. Remember to alternate feet.

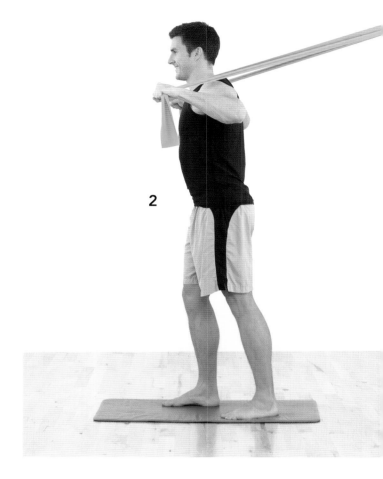

2

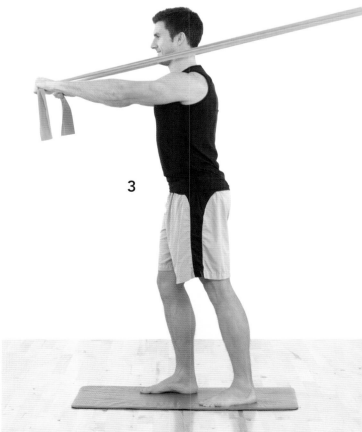

3

Chest fly

This exercise strengthens your chest and shoulder muscles, giving you great benefits in many sports.

1 Using a resistance band anchor, attach the resistance band securely to a locked door at shoulder level. If using handles, make sure they are securely attached to the ends of the resistance band.

2 Stand with your back towards the anchor point. Keep your feet shoulder-width apart, but with one foot slightly in front of the other, and knees slightly bent. Start the exercise holding the ends of the resistance band at shoulder level. Bend your elbows slightly and lock them in this position, keeping your thumbs upwards and your arms slightly in front of you. Make sure the band is taut.

3 Pull the band inwards, so your palms are facing each other. Hold this position for a count of one, then return to the start position slowly and with control.

Variations

Change the height of the attachment point of the band to a lower anchor point for an inclined chest fly, or a higher anchor point for a declined chest fly. To work your core stability, perform the exercise standing on one leg, and for an additional challenge place a foam- or air-filled stability pad under your foot. Remember to alternate feet.

TIP

Remember to activate your core muscles by sucking in your stomach while exhaling, and when you feel your stomach muscles contract, lock them into this contracted position and continue to breathe normally.

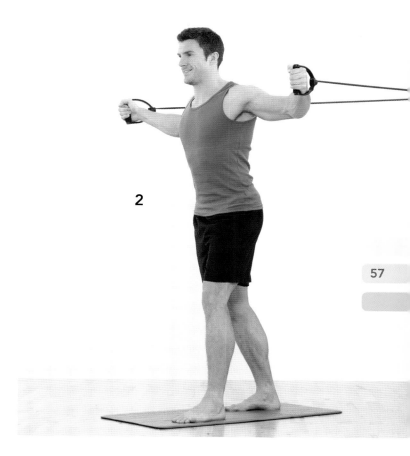

2

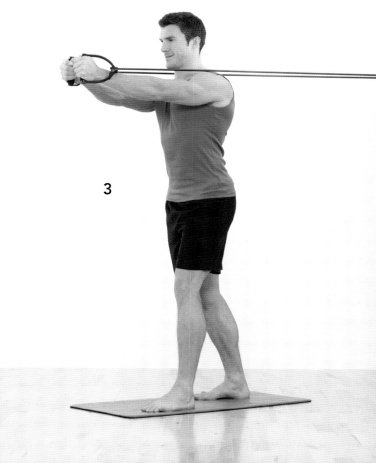

3

Chest pull over

This is a great all-round exercise that focuses on your chest, shoulders and back muscles.

1 Using a resistance band anchor, attach the resistance band securely to a locked door at low level. If using handles, make sure they are securely attached to the ends of the resistance band.

2 Lie on your back on the floor with your head towards the anchor point. Bend your knees and place your feet flat on the floor. Clasp the handles with your arms extended overhead. Slightly bend your elbows and lock them in this position. Keep your thumbs facing each other and ensure that the band is taut. Pull the resistance band down towards your hips. Do not hold your breath at any point. Hold this position for a count of one, then release to the start position slowly and with control.

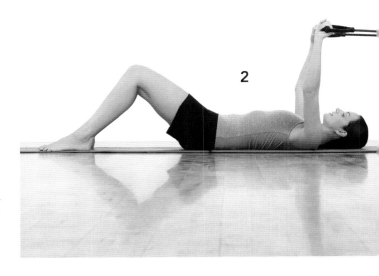

2

VISUALIZATION

Visualizing before executing the techniques for real assists your ability to do the exercise correctly. Perform the technique through your eyes, adding feeling. When you visualize, ensure your technique is absolutely perfect. Practise your visualizing when exercising, then expand it into other areas of your training.

CAUTION

Do not arch your back or lift your hips. Keep your arms moving at the same rate during both phases of the exercise.

2

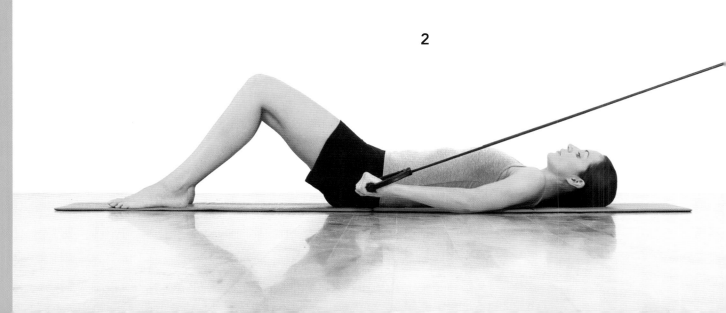

Push up

A simply wonderful exercise for strengthening your chest, upper arms, back and core muscles.

TARGET HEART RATE

Are you training within your target heart rate? Time your heartbeat for 15 seconds. Start counting the first beat that falls on zero seconds as follows 0-1-2-3... . At 15 seconds, multiply the number of beats by four. This will give you your beats per minute.

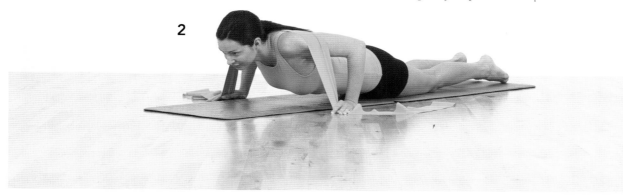

1 Lie chest-down on the floor. Pass the resistance band across your back and wrap it around both hands so that you can place your palms flat on the floor at shoulder level, and slightly more than shoulder-width apart. Make sure the band is taut. Stretch out your legs with your feet together. Look slightly forwards rather than at the floor, so that you are resting on your chin rather than your nose. Make sure your core muscles are activated by sucking in your stomach while exhaling and when you feel your stomach muscles contract, lock them into this contracted position and continue to breathe normally.

2 Straighten your arms, pushing your body off the floor slowly as you exhale steadily. Keep your upper and lower back straight, correcting any arching. Hold this position for a count of one, then release very slowly to the start position, inhaling all the way.

TIP

This exercise can be performed while kneeling to reduce the tension, enabling more repetitions.

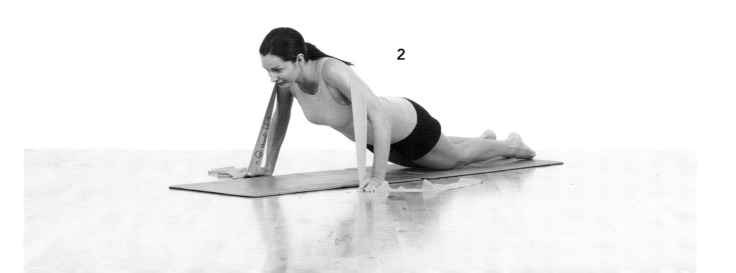

Latissimus dorsi pull down

Try to maintain a smooth and controlled action throughout this exercise's full range of motion.

1 Using a resistance band anchor, attach the resistance band securely at the top of a locked door. Stand facing the anchor point with your feet shoulder width apart, then place one foot slightly in front of the other, with your knees slightly bent.

2 Clasp one end of the resistance band in each hand with your elbows extended out in front of you above shoulder height, thumbs upwards. Make sure the resistance band is taut – move further away from the anchor point if necessary.

3 Activate your core muscles, then slowly pull the resistance band handles back and down, bending at the elbows and continuing through until your hands are by your sides, thumbs to your body. Pause in this position for a count of one, then slowly and with control return to the start position.

Variation
Maintain extended arms throughout the action from start to end, but do not lock out your elbows – bend the elbows slightly and then lock them in this soft position.

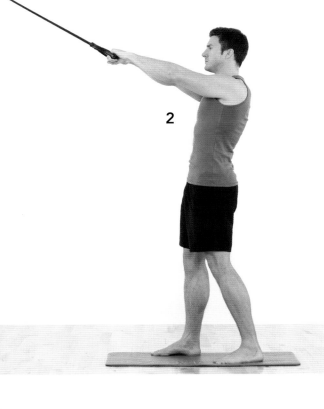

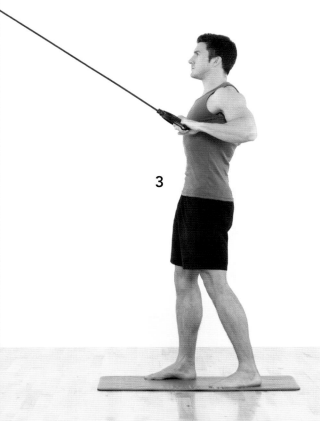

TIP

Maintain a straight back and neck throughout – do not arch your back or roll your shoulders forwards.

Seated row

This exercise works your shoulders, arms, back and core muscle groups, giving them a great work out.

1 Sit on the floor with your legs extended. The resistance band can either be securely anchored at low level, or simply looped under both feet. You can increase or decrease the resistance depending on where you grasp the band. Make sure there is equal resistance in both hands.

2 Activate your core muscles by sucking in your stomach while exhaling, and, when you feel your stomach muscles contract, lock them into this contracted position and continue to breathe normally.

3 Begin to pull your arms back towards your torso, bending your elbows and tucking your arms into your sides. Continue pulling until your hands reach your abdominal area; hold this position for a count of one. The exercise is only half complete, so maintain your concentration and breathing. Do not arch your lower back – keep it straight and maintain the tension in your core muscles.

4 Release slowly and with control to the start position, using your arms – do not bend forwards to complete the motion.

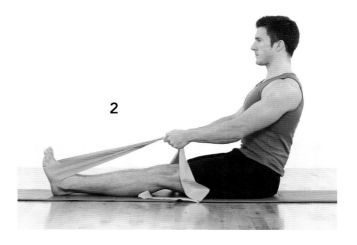

2

TIP

If your hands begin to sweat from holding the resistance band, slowly release the tension and then dry your hands and the band using a towel. Letting go of a fully tensioned band can be dangerous.

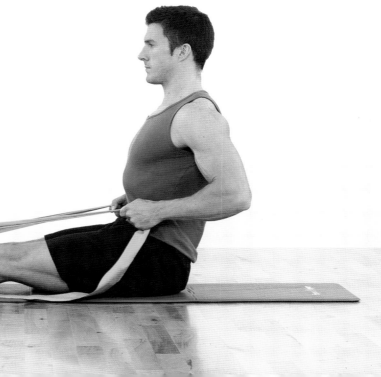

3

Shoulder shrug

This exercise for improving your upper back strength will assist you in anything from windsurfing to carrying heavy bags of shopping.

1 Stand with your left foot in the middle of your looped band, your right foot comfortably spaced behind your left foot and your knees slightly bent.

2 Clasp one end of the resistance band in each hand. If using handles, make sure they are securely attached to the ends of the band. With your arms by your sides and both elbows straight, the resistance band should be taut; if it is not taut, either grip the band further down its length, or, if using handles, shorten the length of the band.

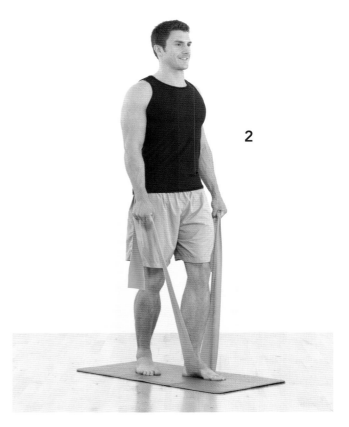

3 With your thumbs inwards, towards your body, lift your shoulders upwards. Make sure you do not bend your elbows – keep them extended. Maintain a straight back and avoid arching your neck – keep it straight throughout the exercise. When your shoulders are in a full shrug, hold the position for a count of one, then return to the start position slowly and with control. Keep your core muscles activated throughout the exercise.

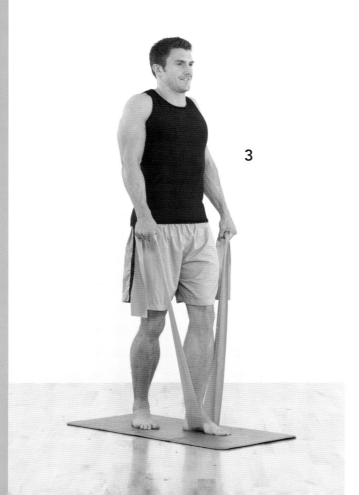

TIP

To work your core stability, perform the exercise while standing on one leg; for an additional challenge place a foam- or air-filled stability pad under your foot. Alternate the leg you stand on during core stability, completing half your repetitions on each leg.

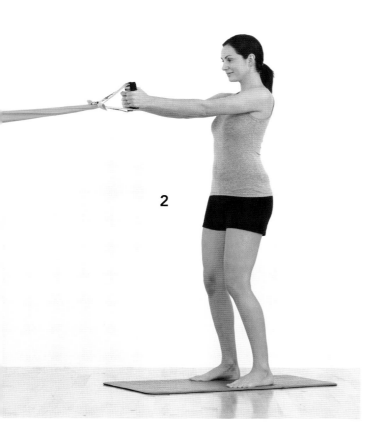

2

Reverse fly

When performing this exercise, you will feel the demands on your muscles increase as you go through the whole motion.

1 Using a resistance band anchor, attach the resistance band securely to a locked door at shoulder level. If using handles, make sure they are securely attached to the ends of the resistance band.

2 Stand facing towards the anchor point. Keep your feet shoulder-width apart, but with the left foot slightly in front of the right, and knees slightly bent. Hold one end of the resistance band in each hand, with your arms extended out in front of you at shoulder level. Bend your elbows slightly and lock them in this position, keeping your thumbs upwards and making sure the band is taut. Move further away from the anchor point to increase the tension of the resistance band and move closer to reduce the tension.

3 Pull the band outwards, until your arms are in a straight line with your shoulders. Hold this position for a count of one, then return to the start position slowly and with control. Half way through your repetitions, swap feet so that the right foot is in front of the left.

Variations
Change the height of the attachment point of the resistance band to a lower anchor point for an inclined reverse fly, or a higher anchor point for a declined reverse fly. Additionally you can work your core while standing on one leg, and for an additional challenge place a foam- or air-filled stability pad under your foot. Remember to alternate feet.

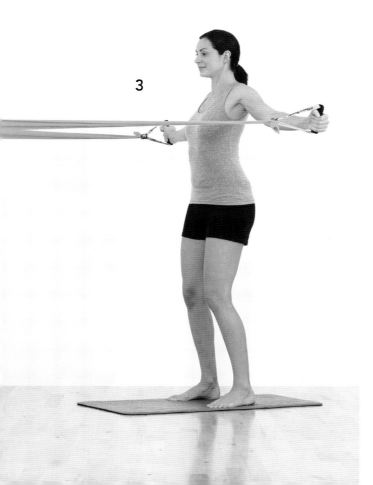

3

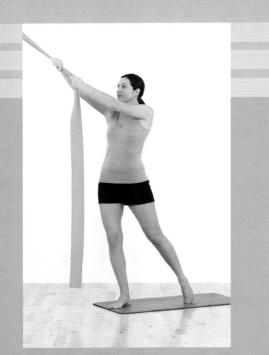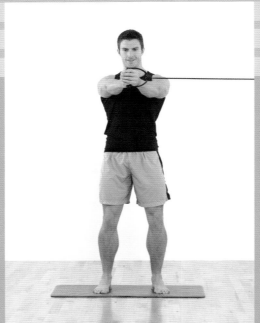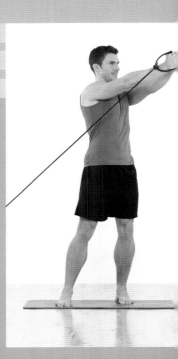

5

abdominal and lower back exercises

The abdominals and lower back muscles are collectively known as the 'core'. 'Core stability' is the ability to control the position and movement of the central portion of the body. Unless stated otherwise in this book, you are required to activate your abdominal muscles when exercising with the resistance band. This activation stabilizes your body while strengthening your core at the same time. Strengthening the abdominals and lower back muscles helps reduce the risk of injury from bad posture and improves the foundation for all arm and leg movements. In addition, strengthening the abdominals and lower back can prevent and improve lower back pain. Increasing your core stability is beneficial for all types of sports and physical activities.

Standing trunk twist

A simple and highly effective exercise that targets your torso and your core muscles. It can help you in activities ranging from digging and raking to rugby and rowing.

1 Using a resistance band anchor, attach the resistance band securely to a locked door at shoulder level. If using a handle, make sure it is securely attached to the end of the resistance band.

2 Stand with your left side towards the anchor point. Position your left foot slightly in front of the right, shoulder-width apart and knees slightly bent. Hold the end of the resistance band in both hands, with your arms extended out in front of you at shoulder level. Bend your elbows slightly and lock them in this position, keeping your thumbs upwards and making sure the band is taut. Move further away from the anchor point to increase the tension of the resistance band and move closer to reduce the tension. Activate your core muscles and hold the contraction throughout the exercise.

3 Slowly rotate your trunk away from the anchor point, keeping your arms braced in the same position. Hold the end position for a count of one, then return to the start position slowly and with control.

4 Reverse your position to work the other side.

Variation

To work your core stability, perform the exercise standing on one leg, and for an additional challenge place a foam- or air-filled stability pad under your foot. Remember to alternate feet.

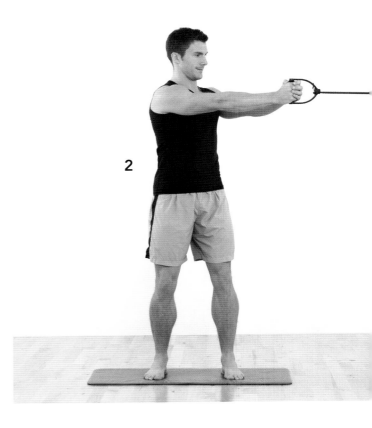

2

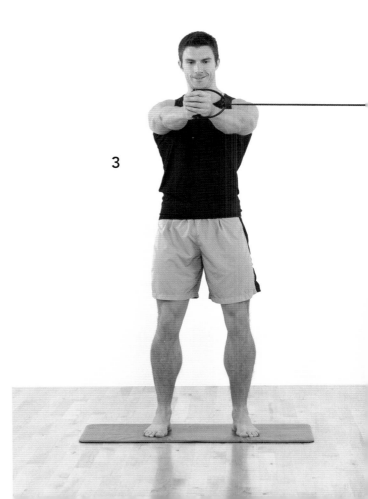

3

Twisting trunk curl

This intensive abdominal exercise will improve your core strength, help you to improve your posture and possibly help reduce lower back pain.

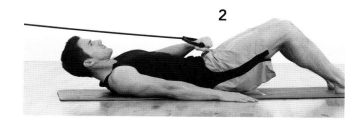

2

1 Using a resistance band anchor, attach the resistance band securely to a locked door at low level. Lie on your back with your head towards the anchor point and slightly to the right of it. Bend your knees and keep your feet flat on the floor. Use a padded mat for additional comfort. For stability throughout the exercise, rest your right arm on the floor, extended at an angle from your side.

2 Clasp the end of the resistance band in your left hand, palm downwards. Extend your left arm in front of you and across your torso towards your right hip, maintaining a slight bend at your elbow. Make sure the resistance band is taut. Activate your core muscles and exhale as you lift your head slightly and stretch your arm further across to your right side, aiming your left hand towards the outside of your body, as if you were folding your left shoulder to your right hip. This should be a smooth all-in-one-action – do not lift first then turn sideways.

3 When you have reached the end of your curl, pause for a count of one, then inhale as you curl back down to the start position.

4 Reverse your position to work the other side.

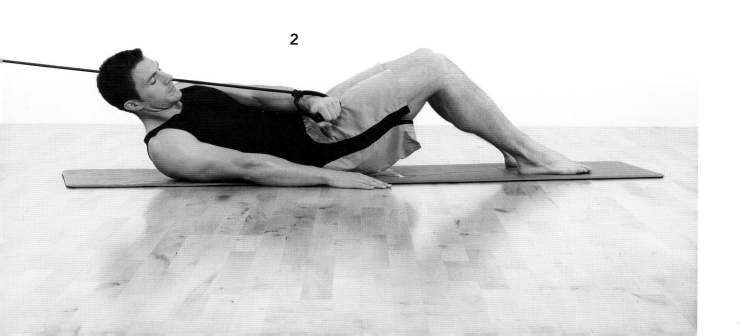

2

Crunch

This exercise tones your abdominal muscles and improves your core stability.

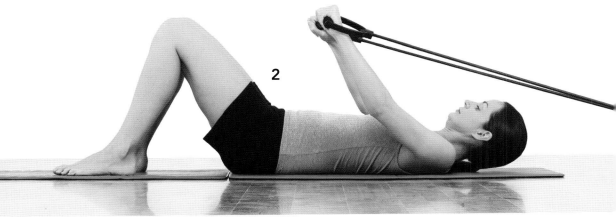

2

1 Using a resistance band anchor, attach the resistance band securely to a locked door at low level. Lie on your back with your head towards the anchor point, bend your knees and place your feet flat on the floor. Use a padded mat for additional comfort.

2 Clasp the ends of the resistance band in both hands, palms downwards. Extend your arms out in front of you, maintaining a slight bend at your elbows. Ensure the resistance band is taut. Imagine there is a tennis ball under your chin, and hold this image throughout the exercise to prevent your chin from touching your chest.

3 Activate your core muscles and exhale as you lift your head, looking forwards towards your thighs, and curl your trunk upwards, lifting your shoulder blades from the floor. This should be a smooth action – do not jerk or bounce up.

4 When you have reached the end of your curl, pause for a count of one, then breathe in as you curl back down to the start position.

3

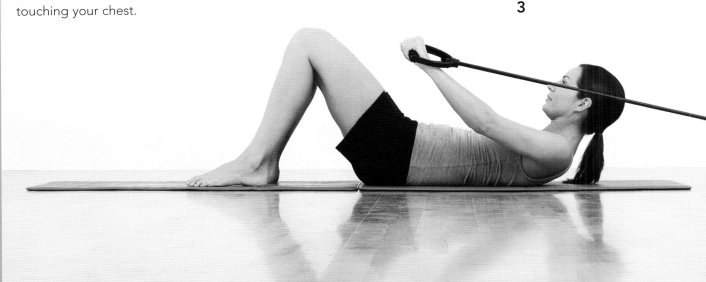

Abdominal crunch

If you do this exercise correctly, you'll feel the tension in the lower region of your abdomen.

TARGET HEART RATE

Are you training within your target heart rate? Time your heartbeat for 15 seconds. Start counting the first beat that falls on zero seconds as follows 0-1-2-3... . At 15 seconds, multiply the number of beats by four. This will give you your beats per minute.

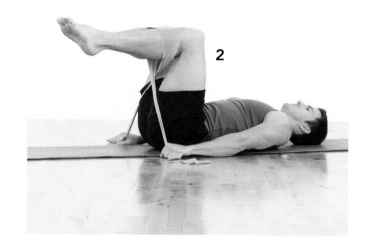

TIP

To reap the full benefit of this exercise, maintain control of the movement throughout and take your time – there is no rush. Do not lift your head or shoulders.

1 Lie on your back, on a padded mat for additional comfort. Wrap the band's full width around your lower legs, just below your knees. Cross the lengths of resistance band over behind your thighs and hold one end of the band in each hand with your arms on the floor, hands by your hips, palms downwards.

2 Bend your hips to a 90-degree angle and your knees to a 90-degree angle, so your feet are in the air, keeping your back flat on the floor. The resistance band must be taut – adjust your grip to pull the band tighter if necessary.

3 Now, lift your hips off the floor against the resistance of the band and hold for a count of one, then slowly release.

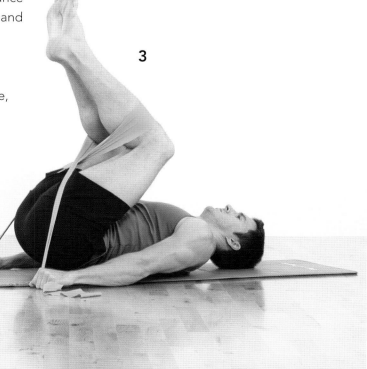

Trunk 'wood chop'

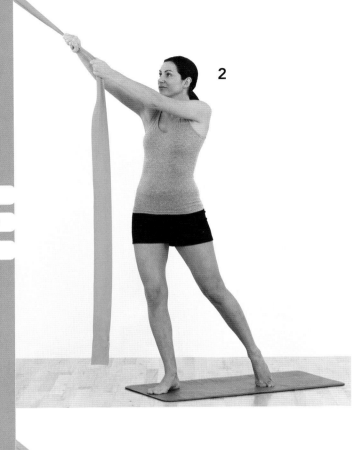

2

This exercise targets your trunk muscles, helping strengthen numerous muscles in your body such as your abs and internal and external oblique muscles.

1 Using a resistance band anchor, attach the resistance band securely to a locked door at high level. If using a handle, make sure it is securely attached to the end of the resistance band.

2 Stand with your right side towards the anchor point. Position your feet shoulder-width apart, with your right foot slightly in front of the left and knees slightly bent. Hold the end of the resistance band with your arms extended high out in front towards the anchor point. Bend your elbows slightly and lock them in this position. Slightly rotate your trunk towards the band, making sure the band is taut. Move further away from the anchor point to increase the tension of the resistance band and move closer to reduce the tension. Activate your core muscles and hold the contraction throughout the exercise.

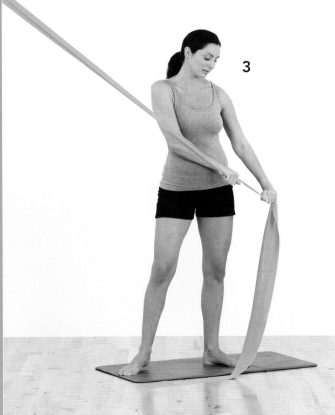

3

3 Pull the resistance band down to your left hip with both hands, slowly rotating your trunk away from the anchor point and keeping your elbows braced in the same position. Hold the end position for a count of one, then return to the start position slowly and with control.

4 Reverse your position to work the opposite side.

Variation
You can stand on your left leg to work your core, and for an additional challenge, place a foam- or air-filled stability pad under your foot. Remember to alternate feet when exercising the opposite side.

Reverse trunk 'wood chop'

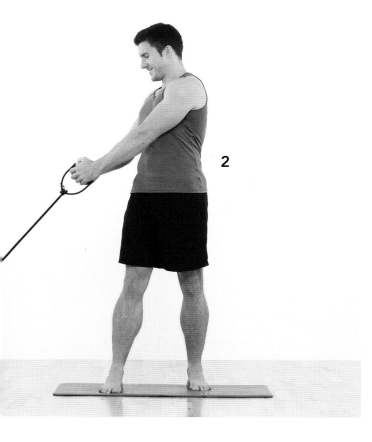

2

The reverse trunk 'wood chop' targets the same muscles as the exercise opposite. For most, the benefits are primarily for sports rather than chopping wood!

1 Using a resistance band anchor, attach the resistance band securely to a locked door at low level. If using a handle, make sure it is securely attached to the end of the resistance band.

2 Stand with your right side towards the anchor point. Position your feet shoulder-width apart, with your right foot slightly in front of the left and knees slightly bent. Hold the end of the resistance band with your arms extended low out in front towards the anchor point. Bend your elbows slightly and lock them in this position. Slightly rotate your trunk towards the band, making sure the band is taut. Move further away from the anchor point to increase the tension of the resistance band and move closer to reduce the tension. Activate your core muscles and hold the contraction throughout the exercise.

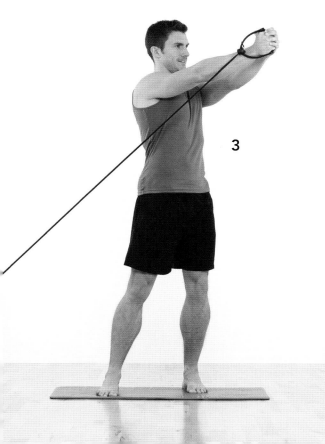

3

3 Pull the resistance band up towards your left shoulder with both hands, slowly rotating your trunk away from the anchor point and keeping your elbows braced in the same position. Hold the end position for a count of one, then return to the start position slowly and with control.

4 Reverse your position to work the opposite side.

Variation
You can stand on your left leg to work your core, and for an additional challenge place a foam- or air-filled stability pad under your foot. Remember to alternate feet when exercising the opposite side.

Side bend

The side bend helps to encourage a good posture.

1 Stand on the middle of the resistance band with your feet shoulder-width apart. Keep your knees and hips slightly bent and your back straight, and make sure the band is secure. Hold one end of the resistance band in each hand.

2 Extend your right arm high above your head with a slightly bent elbow that you lock into this position, and extend your left arm down by your side. Lean your trunk towards the left, stretching the band with your right hand. Hold the end position for a count of one, then return to the start position slowly and with control.

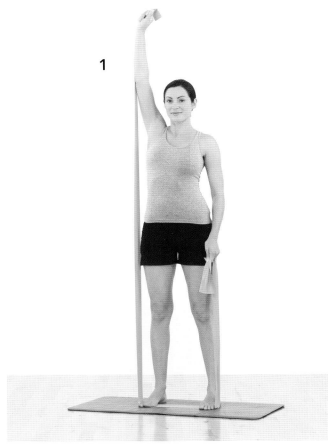

1

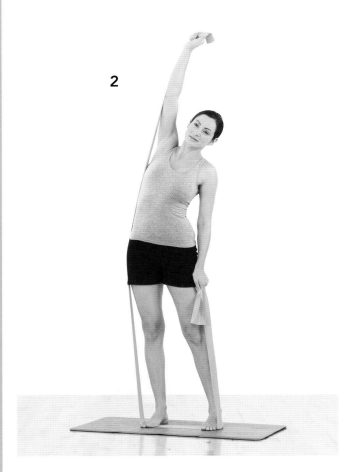

2

3 Reverse your position to work the opposite side.

Variation
You can work your core by standing on your right leg, with one end of the resistance band secured beneath your foot. Hold the other end of the band in your right hand, allowing your left hand to rest by your side. Extend your right arm high above your head with a slightly bent elbow that you lock into this position, and extend your left arm down by your side. Lean your trunk towards the left, stretching the band with your right hand. Hold the end position for a count of one, then return to the start position slowly and with control.

Side bridge

This exercise is difficult, but good for toning the abdominals and the muscles in the side of your trunk.

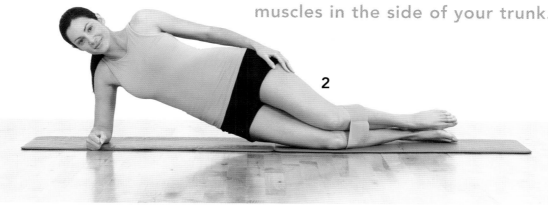

1 Wrap the resistance band around your lower legs, just below your knees, and tie the ends, making sure it is taut. Lie on your right side on the floor, using a padded mat for additional comfort. Bend your right elbow under your right shoulder, propping yourself up off the floor.

2 Activate your core muscles by sucking in your stomach while exhaling, and, when you feel your stomach muscles contract, lock them into this contracted position and continue to breathe normally. Keeping your knees bent, lift your hips up off the floor, maintaining a straight back.

3 Holding this position, separate your knees, causing the resistance band to stretch. Hold this position for a count of one, then return to the start position slowly and with control.

4 Reverse your position to work the opposite side.

VISUALIZATION

Visualizing before executing the techniques for real assists your ability to carry out the exercise correctly. Perform the technique through your eyes, adding feeling. When you visualize, ensure your technique is absolutely perfect. Practise your visualizing when exercising, then expand it into other areas of your training.

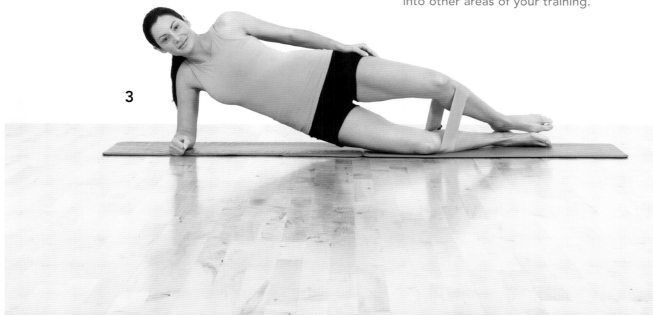

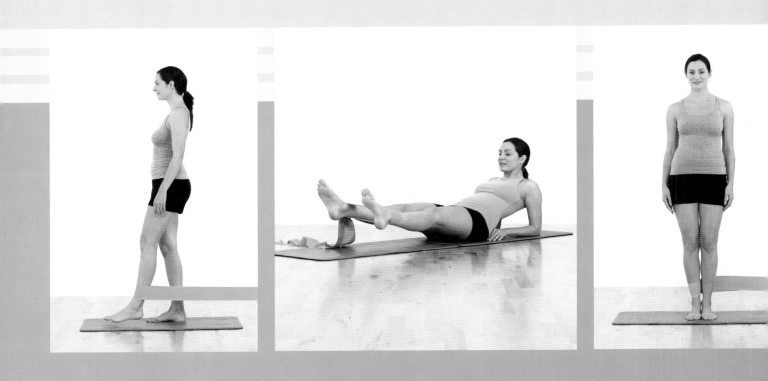

6

hip and thigh exercises

The hip and thigh region is one of the most important areas you can strengthen. Connecting the lower extremities to the trunk, the hips provide a stable base for the 'core'. The hips are fundamental for movement, transferring your centre of gravity during walking and running. The gluteal muscles provide pelvic stability, which is again fundamental during walking and running. Weakness of the gluteal muscles is linked to back pain, knee pain, hip pain and repetitive ankle injuries. Also, imbalances of strength and flexibility between your quadriceps and hamstring muscles can be linked to knee pain. Resistance band exercises for the hips and thighs can assist your everyday activities, particularly walking, as well as improving stability and balance.

Hip flexion

This exercise is very good for helping to develop your hip muscles. These muscles assist you in sitting up and working them helps to maximize the length of your stride when walking or sprinting.

1 Using a resistance band anchor, attach the resistance band securely to a locked door at low level. Tie the loose ends of the band together to form a loop.

2 Stand with your back towards the anchor point and loop the resistance band around the lower left leg, just above your ankle. Keep your back straight and both knees slightly bent, but with your weight balanced on your right leg.

3 Slowly 'kick' your left leg forwards. Hold your leg out in the 'kicked' position for a count of one, then slowly release to the start position.

4 Reverse your position to work the right leg.

TIP

Do not 'kick' from your knee – the 'kick' comes from your hip. Execute the full range of the exercise with a straight back and avoid leaning forwards. For an additional challenge, place a foam- or air-filled stability pad under your right foot.

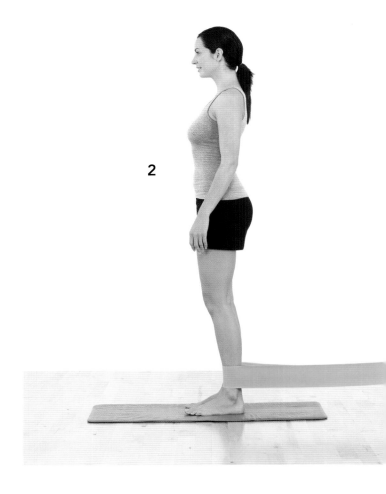

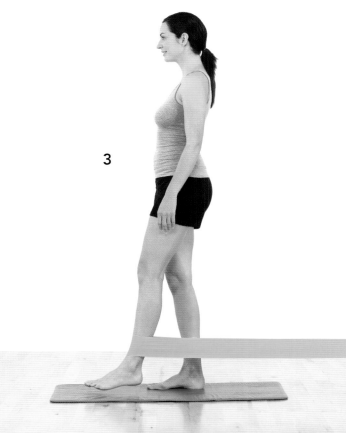

Hip extension

This exercise develops the muscles that assist you with locomotion, the muscles that help you walk, run and climb stairs.

1 Using a resistance band anchor, attach the resistance band securely to a locked door at low level. Tie the loose ends of the band together to form a loop.

2 Standing facing towards the anchor point, loop the resistance band around the lower right leg, just above your ankle. Keep your back straight and both knees slightly bent, but with your weight balanced on your left leg.

3 Slowly 'kick' your right leg backwards. Hold your leg back in the 'kicked' position for a count of one, then slowly release to the start position.

4 Reverse your position to work the opposite side.

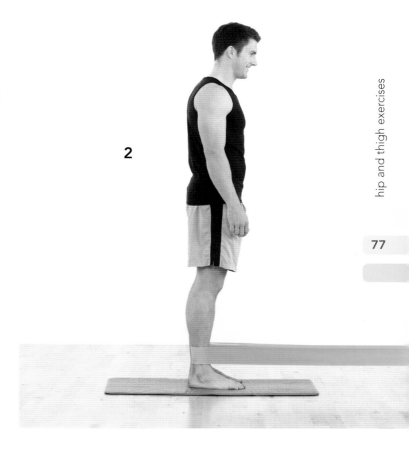

2

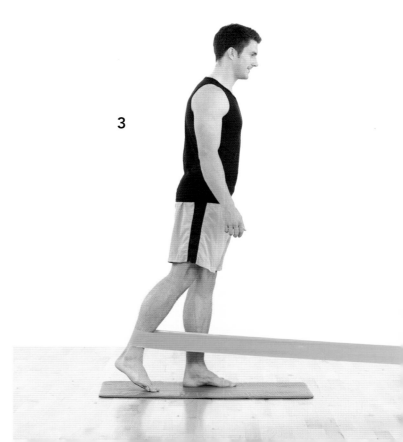

3

Hip abduction (gluteus medius)

This intense exercise is very effective at toning the abdominals and the muscles in the rear and sides of your hip.

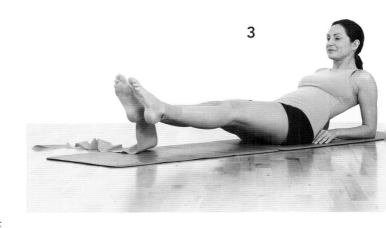

1 Sit on the floor with your legs extended and your knees slightly bent; use a padded floor mat for additional comfort. Loop the resistance band around both legs, just above your ankles, and tie the ends of the band together. Lean back onto your elbows in a reclined position.

2 Activate your core muscles by sucking in your stomach while exhaling, and, when you feel your stomach muscles contract, lock them into this contracted position and continue to breathe normally.

3 Lift both legs off the floor by approximately 10–15 cm (4–6 in). Maintaining your right leg in this position, draw your left leg out to the side, still 10–15 cm (4–6 in) off the floor. Hold this outward draw for a count of one, then slowly release.

4 Repeat, drawing out the right leg.

CAUTION

Never hold your breath when stretching or exercising. Exhaling after a deep breath enables you to release muscle tension in your body. This enables the muscles to relax more and therefore increases their length.

TIP

This is a strenuous exercise. Rest with your legs on the floor in between alternating the 'working' leg.

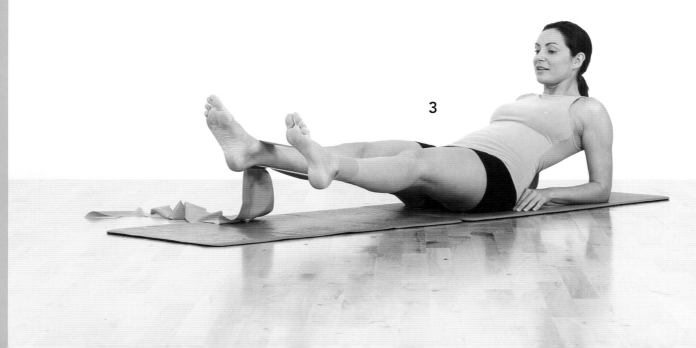

Hip abduction with core emphasis

This exercise is of great benefit if you take part in sports that require a side-step motion such as cross-country skiing and ice skating.

1 Using a resistance band anchor, attach the resistance band securely to a locked door at low level. Tie the loose ends of the resistance band together to form a loop.

2 Standing with your left side towards the anchor point, loop the resistance band around your lower right leg, just above your ankle. The band can pass either in front of you or behind you. Keep your back straight and both knees slightly bent, but with your weight balanced on your right leg.

3 Start with both legs together, making sure the resistance band is taut; adjust the tension by moving further away from the anchor point to increase the tension or closer to reduce it. Slowly draw your right leg outwards to your right side. Hold the outward 'drawn' position for a count of one, then slowly release to the start position.

4 Reverse your position to work the opposite side.

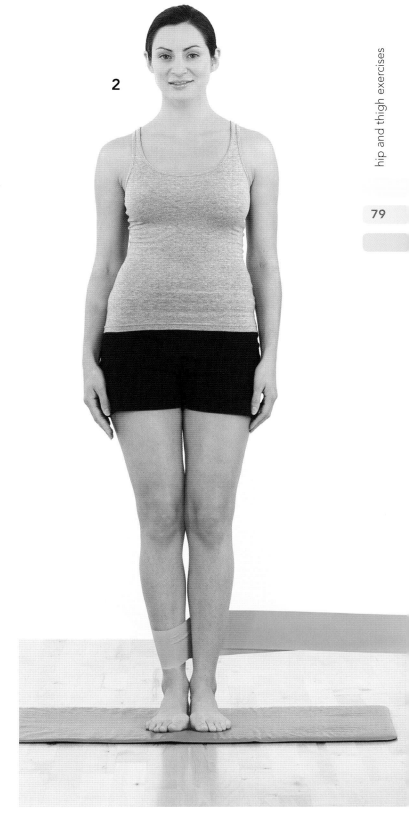

2

TIP

Do not 'draw' from your waist – the movement comes from your hip. Execute the full range of the exercise with a straight back and avoid leaning forwards or to the side.

Hip adduction with core emphasis

Your adductor muscles are located on the inside of your thighs. They are used in anything from horse riding to getting into a car.

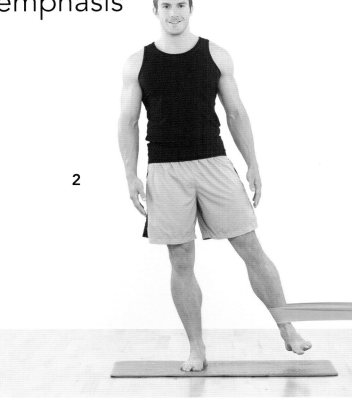

2

1 Using a resistance band anchor, attach the resistance band securely to a locked door at low level. Tie the loose ends of the resistance band together to form a loop.

2 Standing with your left side towards the anchor point, loop the resistance band around your lower left leg, just above your ankle. Keep your back straight and both knees slightly bent, but with your weight balanced on your right leg. Start with your left leg already drawn out to your left side, making sure the resistance band is taut – adjust the tension by moving further away from the anchor point to increase the tension or closer to reduce it.

3 Slowly draw your left leg in towards your right leg, bringing both legs together. Hold your left leg in this position for a count of one, then slowly release to the start position.

4 Reverse your position to work the opposite side.

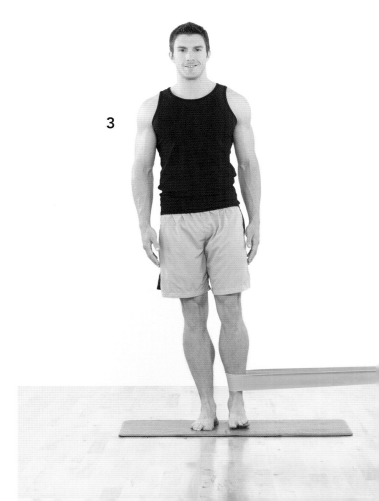

3

TIP

For an additional challenge, place a foam- or air-filled stability pad under your right foot.

Leg press

Strengthening your thigh and buttock muscles can help you in many sports including running, surfing, windsurfing and jumping.

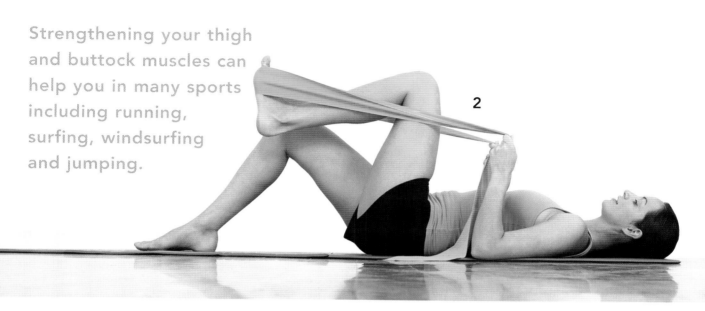

1 Lie on your back with both knees bent; use a padded mat for additional comfort. Loop the middle of the resistance band under your left foot, clasping one end of the band in each hand.

ACTIVATING YOUR CORE

Activate your core muscles by sucking in your stomach while exhaling, and, when you feel your stomach muscles contract, lock them into this contracted position and continue to breathe normally.

2 Keeping your right foot flat on the floor, flex your left hip, raising your left foot and keeping your left knee bent. Ensure the resistance band is taut – adjust your grip on the band to increase or decrease tension.

3 Keeping your back straight and flat on the floor, slowly extend your left knee until your leg is straight. Hold this position for a count of one, then release to the start position slowly and with control.

4 Reverse your position to work the opposite side.

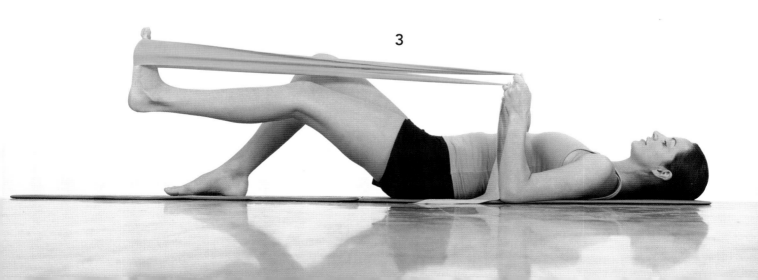

Knee flexion, hamstrings

The hamstrings, a collection of three large muscles located at the rear of each thigh, are the focus of this exercise.

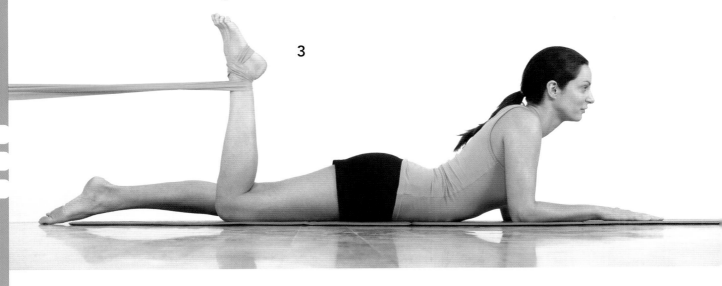

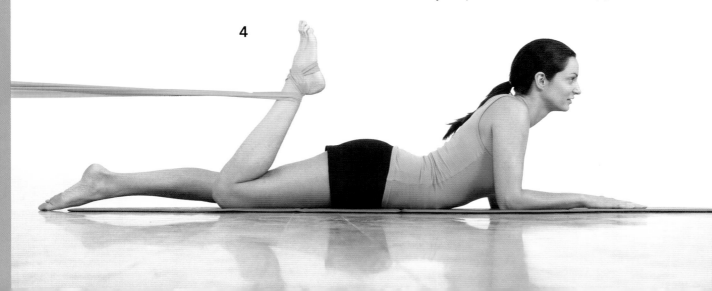

1 Using a resistance band anchor, attach the resistance band securely to a locked door at low level. Tie the loose ends of the resistance band together to form a loop.

2 Lie on your front, using a padded mat for additional comfort, with your head away from the anchor point. Wrap the middle of the resistance band about your right foot and ankle.

3 Bend your right knee to a 90-degree angle, making sure the resistance band is taut. Adjust the tension by moving further away from the anchor point to increase the tension or closer to reduce it.

4 Pull your right foot slowly towards your buttocks. Keep your hips, thighs and stomach on the floor and do not arch your lower back. Hold this position for a count of one with your knee fully flexed, then slowly release your leg back to the start position.

5 Reverse your position to work the opposite side.

Knee extension, quadriceps

This excellent exercise strengthens your quadriceps, the four muscles located at the front of your thighs.

1 Using a resistance band anchor, attach the resistance band securely to a locked door at low level. Tie the loose ends of the resistance band together to form a loop.

2 Lie on your front, using a padded mat for additional comfort, with your head towards the anchor point. Wrap the middle of the resistance band around your right foot and ankle.

3 Bend your right knee to a 90-degree angle, making sure the resistance band is taut. Adjust the

tension by moving further away from the anchor point to increase the tension or closer to reduce it.

4 Push your right foot slowly downwards towards the floor. Keep your hips and stomach on the floor and do not arch your lower back.

5 Hold this position for a count of one with your leg fully extended, then release your leg back to the start position slowly and with control.

6 Reverse your position to work the opposite side.

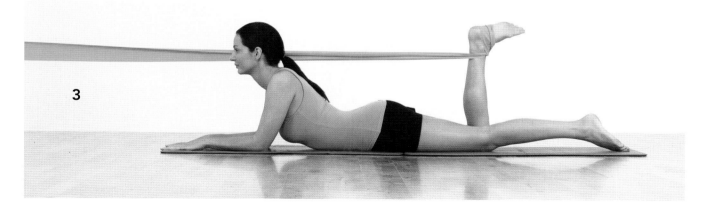

3

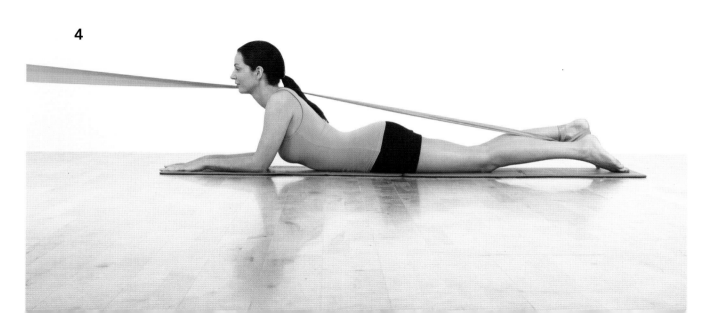

4

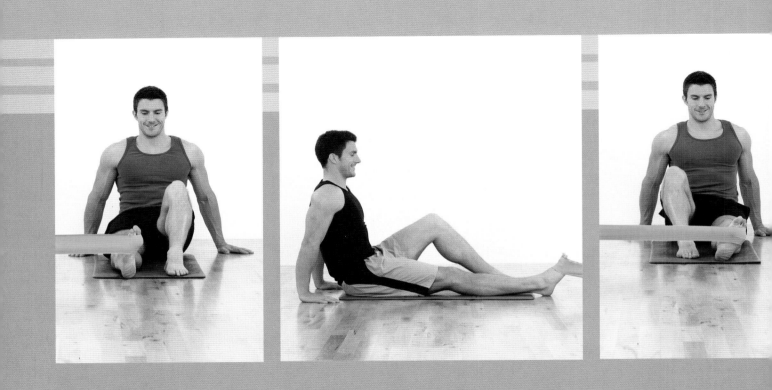

7
lower leg and ankle exercises

The lower leg muscles and ankles have important roles with your stability, locomotion and action within the walking and running cycle, known as 'gait'. Improving your lower leg strength can go a long way towards improving your balance and stability, especially when participating in sports that require quick changes of direction, such as football, tennis and basketball. Resistance band exercises are excellent for strengthening the lower leg and stabilizing your ankles.

Ankle inversion

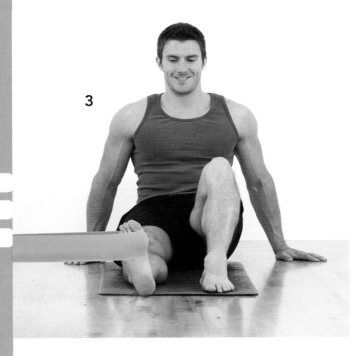

3

Strong ankles improve your balance and stability. Additionally, this exercise will also help to improve your mobility.

1 Using a resistance band anchor, attach the resistance band securely to a locked door at low level. Tie the loose ends of the resistance band together to form a loop.

2 Sit on the floor, using a padded mat for additional comfort, with your right side towards the anchor point, your right leg extended and your right foot directly in line with the anchor point. Loop the resistance band around your right foot.

3 Start with your right foot rotated outwards towards the anchor point, making sure the resistance band is taut. Adjust the tension by moving further away from the anchor point to increase the tension or closer to reduce it.

4 Invert your right foot by rotating it slowly inwards about your ankle. Hold your foot in full inversion for a count of one, then slowly return your foot to the start position. Do not rotate from your leg to complete the motion, maintain your knee in a fixed stable position.

5 Reverse your position to work the opposite side.

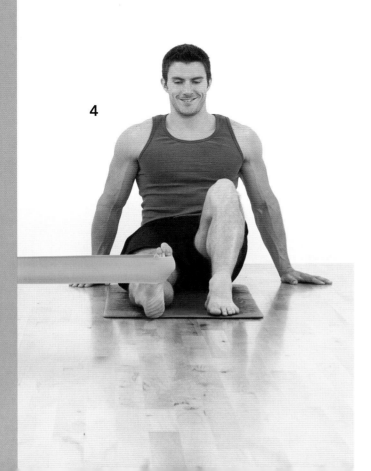

4

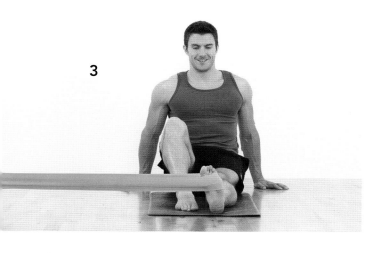

3

Ankle eversion

Strengthening the ankles will help to reduce the chance of suffering ankle, knee and hip injuries. If you do receive one, strong ankles can assist your rehabilitation.

1 Using a resistance band anchor, attach the resistance band securely to a locked door at low level. Tie the loose ends of the resistance band together to form a loop.

2 Sit on the floor, using a padded mat for additional comfort, with your right side towards the anchor point, your left leg extended and your left foot directly in line with the anchor point. Loop the resistance band around your left foot.

3 Start with your left foot rotated towards the anchor point, making sure the resistance band is taut. Adjust the tension by moving further away from the anchor point to increase the tension or closer to reduce it.

4 Evert your left foot by rotating your left foot slowly outwards, rotating about your ankle. Hold your foot in full eversion for a count of one, then slowly return your foot to the start position. Do not rotate from your leg to complete the motion, maintain your knee in a fixed stable position.

5 Reverse your position to work the opposite side.

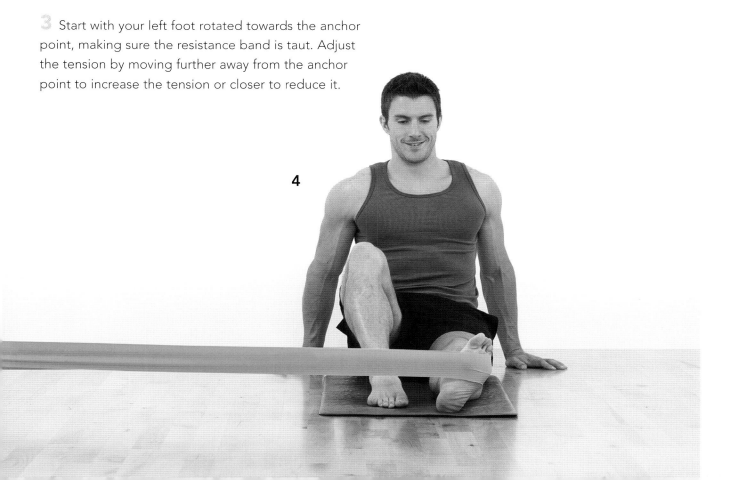

4

Ankle dorsiflexion

This simple and very effective exercise works the muscles that lift your toes, lift your foot and let your foot pivot around your ankle.

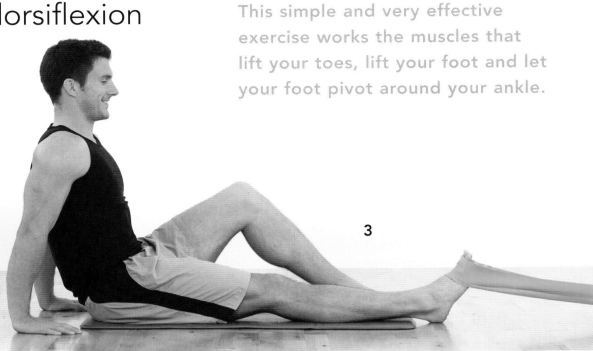

3

1 Using a resistance band anchor, attach the resistance band securely to a locked door at low level. Tie the loose ends of the resistance band together to form a loop.

2 Sit on the floor facing the anchor point, using a padded mat for additional comfort, with your legs extended.

3 Loop the middle of the resistance band over the top of your extended right foot, making sure the resistance band is taut. Adjust the tension by moving further away from the anchor point to increase the tension or closer to reduce it.

4 Flex your ankle towards your head against the resistance band. Hold your ankle in full flexion for a count of one, then slowly return your foot to the start position.

5 Reverse your position to work the opposite side.

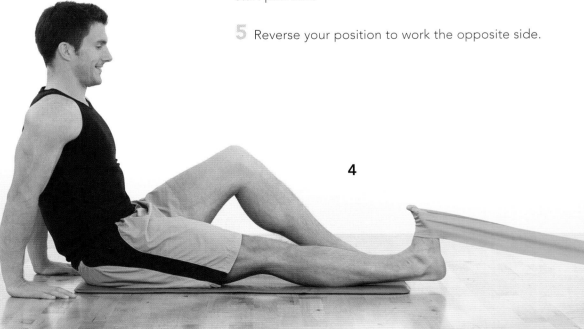

4

Ankle planterflexion

This is an excellent ankle exercise, working all the muscles in your lower leg that assist in pushing your foot downwards.

1 Sit on the floor with your legs extended, using a padded mat for additional comfort. Loop the middle of the resistance band under your right foot and clasp one end of the band in each hand.

2 Start with your right ankle flexed, making sure the resistance band is taut. If necessary, adjust your grip on the band, increasing or decreasing the tension accordingly.

3 Extend your ankle away from your head against the resistance band. Hold your ankle in full extension for a count of one, then slowly return your foot to the start position.

4 Reverse your position to work the opposite side.

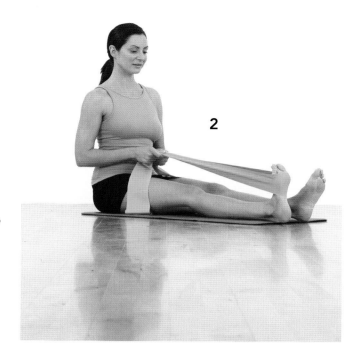

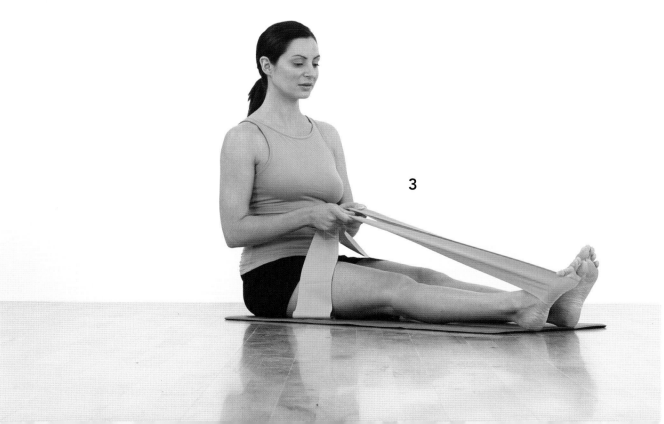

The following pages contain two exercise charts, which between them cover every exercise described in this book. Start your first session with Exercise Chart 1 and your next session with Exercise Chart 2, and continue to alternate for balance and interest.

The exercise charts on the following pages can be used as a guide. You can develop any combination of exercises and use your imagination to develop your own. Remember to balance the exercises – for example, balance your biceps brachii by exercising your triceps brachii, and balance your quadriceps by exercising your hamstrings.

Before you can start your workout you must assess your body type (see pages 18–19). Remember that body type is not how much fat or muscle your body has – it simply means where on your body it would be evident that weight is being added or lost. Once you have decided upon your body type, use the following key to see how you should approach each exercise.

L Represents low-resistance aerobic exercise at high repetitions, ie 20–25 repetitions, completing 2–3 sets. Aerobic exercise increases your heart rate, but you should remain within your Target Heart Rate and not enter into the anaerobic zone.

H Represents higher resistance anaerobic exercise at low repetitions, ie 6–8 repetitions, completing 2–3 sets. Anaerobic exercise adds to muscle bulk, using muscles in a brief, high-intensity activity where oxygen requirements cannot meet the demand of the activity, increasing the breathing and heart rate very quickly and causing fatigue. Remain within your target heart rate and never exceed your maximum heart rate.

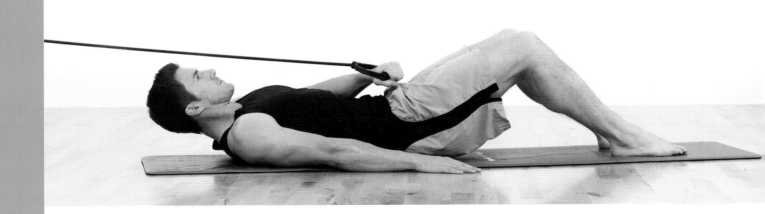

pulling it all together

Always use a low-tension resistance band when you do a new exercise for the first time. This will enable you to achieve the correct technique, and you can then increase the band's resistance if it suits your needs and body type. The low-tension resistance band is also the best band for aerobic exercising and weight loss. Use a higher-tension resistance band for more anaerobic exercises once you have mastered them using a low-tension resistance band.

If you are overweight, reduce the resistance of the exercise and increase the number of repetitions, as fat will be pushed outward as muscle is built.

Always warm up and stretch before you start exercising. Warm down after exercising by gentle jogging on the spot. Warming down enables your heart rate and breathing to return to normal gently after the exertion of exercise.

Remember to work out the target heart rate you will be exercising within (see pages 20–21), and keep a track of your heart rate during your workout.

Do plan ahead, set time aside during your week to exercise. Remember why you are exercising and your desired results. You can make it happen – above all, be consistent with your exercising and be positively motivated (see pages 22–23).

Above all, enjoy the whole process of exercising with resistance bands – they are one of the most useful and versatile exercising tools.

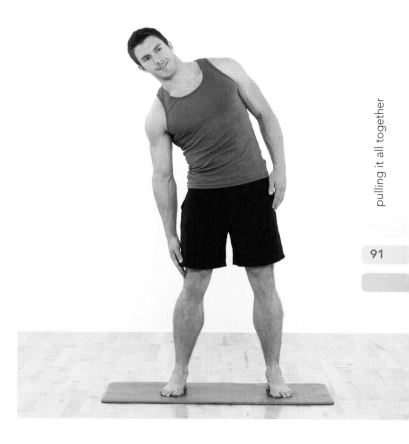

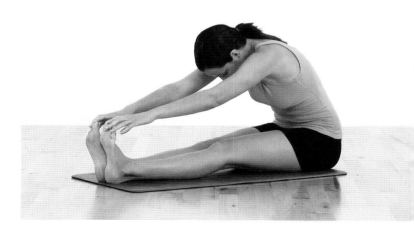

exercise chart 1

Body types (see pages 18–19)	X	Y	I	A
Over shoulder press (page 44)	L	L	H*	H*
Shoulder lateral raise (page 45)	L	L	H*	H*
Shoulder internal rotation (page 48)	L	L	H*	H*
Shoulder external rotation (page 48)	L	L	H*	H*
Wrist forearm pronation (page 52)	L	L	H*	H*
Wrist forearm supination (page 53)	L	L	H*	H*
Chest pull over (page 58)	L	L	H*	H*
Push up (page 59)	L	L	H*	H*
Seated row (page 61)	L	L	H*	H*
Shoulder shrug (page 62)	L	L	H*	H*
Crunch (page 68)	L	L	H*	H*

Abdominal crunch (page 69)	Side bend (page 72)	Side bridge (page 73)	Hip flexion (page 76)	Hip extension (page 77)	Hip adduction with core emphasis (page 80)	Leg press (page 81)	Ankle dorsiflexion (page 88)	Ankle planterflexion (page 89)
L	L	L	L	L	L	L	L	L
L	L	L	H*	H*	H*	H*	H*	H*
H*	H*	H*	H*	H*	H*	H*	H*	H*
H*	H*	H*	L	L	L	L	L	L

L Aerobic exercise
Use a low-tension resistance band with high repetitions, ie 20–25 repetitions, maintaining an increased heart rate, but not entering into the anaerobic zone.

H Anaerobic exercise
Use a high-tension resistance band enabling only low repetitions, ie 6–8 repetitions before you feel fatigue, to add to your muscle bulk.

*   If overweight, use a low-tension resistance band with high repetitions, ie 20–25 repetitions, maintaining an increased heart rate, and not entering into the anaerobic zone.

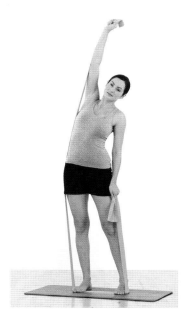

exercise chart 2

Body types (see pages 18–19)	Shoulder diagonal flexion (page 46)	Shoulder diagonal extension (page 47)	Triceps pull-down (page 49)	Biceps curl (page 50)	Wrist curl (page 51)	Reverse wrist curl (page 51)	Standing bench press (page 56)	Chest fly (page 57)	Latissmus dorsi pull down (page 60)	Reverse fly (page 63)	Standing trunk twist (page 66)
X	L	L	L	L	L	L	L	L	L	L	L
Y	L	L	L	L	L	L	L	L	L	L	L
I	H*	H*	H*	H*	H*	H*	H*	H*	H*	H*	H*
A	H*	H*	H*	H*	H*	H*	H*	H*	H*	H*	H*

	Twisting trunk curl (page 67)	Trunk 'wood chop' (page 70)	Reverse trunk 'wood chop' (page 71)	Hip abduction (gluteus medius) (page 78)	Hip abduction with core emphasis (page 79)	Knee flexion, hamstrings (page 82)	Knee extension, quadriceps (page 83)	Ankle inversion (page 86)	Ankle eversion (page 87)
	L	L	L	L	L	L	L	L	L
	L	L	L	H*	H*	H*	H*	H*	H*
	H*	H*	H*	H*	H*	H*	H*	H*	H*
	H*	H*	H*	L	L	L	L	L	L

L Aerobic exercise

Use a low-tension resistance band with high repetitions, ie 20–25 repetitions, maintaining an increased heart rate, but not entering into the anaerobic zone.

H Anaerobic exercise

Use a high-tension resistance band enabling only low repetitions, ie 6–8 repetitions before you feel fatigue, to add to your muscle bulk.

*   If overweight, use a low-tension resistance band with high repetitions, ie 20–25 repetitions, maintaining an increased heart rate, and not entering into the anaerobic zone.

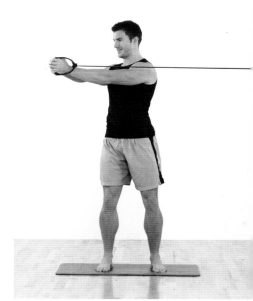

index